Managing chronic conditions

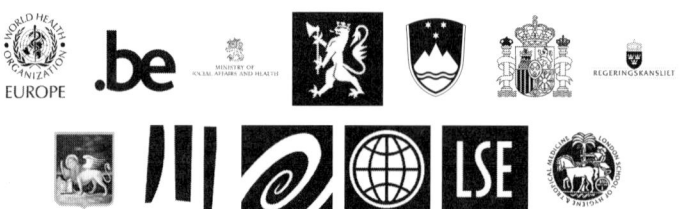

The European Observatory on Health Systems and Policies supports and promotes evidence-based health policy-making through comprehensive and rigorous analysis of health systems in Europe. It brings together a wide range of policy-makers, academics and practitioners to analyse trends in health reform, drawing on experience from across Europe to illuminate policy issues.

The European Observatory on Health Systems and Policies is a partnership between the World Health Organization Regional Office for Europe, the Governments of Belgium, Finland, Norway, Slovenia, Spain and Sweden, the Veneto Region of Italy, the European Investment Bank, the Open Society Institute, the World Bank, the London School of Economics and Political Science and the London School of Hygiene & Tropical Medicine.

Managing chronic conditions
Experience in eight countries

Ellen Nolte

Cécile Knai

Martin McKee

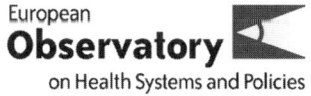

Keywords:

CHRONIC DISEASE - prevention and control
DISEASE MANAGEMENT
DELIVERY OF HEALTH CARE - organization and administration
DENMARK
FRANCE
GERMANY
THE NETHERLANDS
SWEDEN
UNITED KINGDOM
AUSTRALIA
CANADA
EUROPE

© World Health Organization 2008, on behalf of the European Observatory on Health Systems and Policies

All rights reserved. The European Observatory on Health Systems and Policies welcomes requests for permission to reproduce or translate its publications, in part or in full.

> Address requests about publications to: Publications, WHO Regional Office for Europe, Scherfigsvej 8 DK-2100 Copenhagen Ø, Denmark
>
> Alternatively, complete an online request form for documentation, health information, or for permission to quote or translate, on the Regional Office web site (http://www.euro.who.int/pubrequest).

The designations employed and the presentation of the material in this publication do not imply the expression of any opinion whatsoever on the part of the European Observatory on Health Systems and Policies concerning the legal status of any country, territory, city or area or of its authorities, or concerning the delimitation of its frontiers or boundaries. Dotted lines on maps represent approximate border lines for which there may not yet be full agreement.

The mention of specific companies or of certain manufacturers' products does not imply that they are endorsed or recommended by the European Observatory on Health Systems and Policies in preference to others of a similar nature that are not mentioned. Errors and omissions excepted, the names of proprietary products are distinguished by initial capital letters.

All reasonable precautions have been taken by the European Observatory on Health Systems and Policies to verify the information contained in this publication. However, the published material is being distributed without warranty of any kind, either express or implied. The responsibility for the interpretation and use of the material lies with the reader. In no event shall the European Observatory on Health Systems and Policies be liable for damages arising from its use. The views expressed by authors, editors, or expert groups do not necessarily represent the decisions or the stated policy of the European Observatory on Health Systems and Policies.

ISBN 978 92 890 4294 9

Printed in the European Union

Contents

List of tables, figures and boxes	vi
List of abbreviations	ix
Foreword	xiii
Acknowledgements	xv
List of contributors	xvi

1 Managing chronic conditions: 1
   An introduction to the experience in eight countries
   Ellen Nolte, Martin McKee, Cécile Knai

2 Denmark 15
   Michaela Schiøtz, Anne Frølich, Allan Krasnik

3 England 29
   Debra de Silva, Daragh Fahey

4 France 55
   Isabelle Durand-Zaleski, Olivier Obrecht

5 Germany 75
   Ulrich Siering

6 The Netherlands 97
   Eveline Klein Lankhorst, Cor Spreeuwenberg

7 Sweden 115
   Ingvar Karlberg

8 Australia 131
   Nicholas Glasgow, Nicholas Zwar, Mark Harris, Iqbal Hasan, Tanisha Jowsey

9 Canada 161
   Izzat Jiwani, Carl-Ardy Dubois

List of tables, figures and boxes

Tables

Table 2.1	Chronic disease management in Denmark: strengths and weaknesses	26
Table 3.1	Critical success factors for chronic disease programmes in England	46
Table 3.2	Chronic disease management in England: strengths and weaknesses	49
Table 4.1	List of long-term disease (ALD) conditions	58
Table 4.2	Chronic disease management in France: strengths and weaknesses	71
Table 5.1	Criteria for coordinating care levels in the diabetes disease management programme	79
Table 5.2	Chronic disease management in Germany: strengths and weaknesses	92
Table 6.1	Chronic disease management in the Netherlands: strengths and weaknesses	111
Table 7.1	Chronic disease management in Sweden: strengths and weaknesses	126
Table 8.1	Chronic disease management programmes and strategies across states	139
Table 8.2	Chronic disease management in Australia: strengths and weaknesses	153
Table 9.1	Cancer Care Ontario: strengths and weaknesses	176

Figures

Fig. 3.1	The National Health Service and Social Care Long-Term Conditions Model	31
Fig. 3.2	A patient journey in England	37

List of tables, figures and boxes **vii**

Fig. 4.1	Follow-up protocol for insulin therapy	62
Fig. 4.2	Patient journey in a diabetes health network	63
Fig. 5.1	Time line for the introduction of disease management programmes in Germany	78
Fig. 6.1	Care levels in the Matador programme	100
Fig. 8.1	Divisions of General Practice with chronic disease-focused programmes or activities, 2002–2003 to 2004–2005	138
Fig. 8.2	General practitioners' claims for chronic disease initiatives, July 2005 to October 2006	140
Fig. 8.3	Service Incentive Payment claims made by general practitioners in Australia for Asthma 3+, diabetes and mental health from November 2001 to October 2006	141

Boxes

Box 2.1	Cooperating partners within the Østerbro health care centre	19
Box 2.2	Goals for the supplementary training of nurses in diabetes care	23
Box 2.3	Evaluating the rehabilitation programme at Østerbro health care centre	24
Box 3.1	East Sussex "Independence First" Partnerships for Older People Projects	34
Box 3.2	Standards for the National Service Framework for diabetes	39
Box 3.3	Domains of reward in the Quality and Outcomes Framework	43
Box 4.1	Costing patient care in health networks	66
Box 4.2	National audit of health networks	67
Box 4.3	Components of the Chronic Care Model in the French system	68
Box 5.1	Formal development of disease management programmes in Germany	80
Box 5.2	Quality targets in disease management programmes	85

Box 5.3	Formal evaluation criteria of disease management programmes in Germany	88
Box 6.1	Financing arrangements for diabetes care in the Matador programme	106
Box 6.2	Evaluating the Matador programme	109
Box 7.1	Examples of typical care pathways for patients with diabetes, stroke, dementia and mental illness in Sweden	118
Box 7.2	Reforming care for older people	119
Box 7.3	Nurse-led clinics in Sweden	120
Box 7.4	Regional oncology centres in Sweden	122
Box 7.5	Care for those with mental illness	123
Box 8.1	Organization and financing of care planning	135
Box 8.2	Aboriginal and Torres Strait Islanders initiatives	137
Box 8.3	Evaluating the Australian Asthma 3+ Visit Plan	149
Box 9.1	The Western Health Information Collaborative	164
Box 9.2	Community care coordinators in Calgary Health Region	166
Box 9.3	Electronic Health Record system (NetCare) in Edmonton health region	166
Box 9.4	Health and social services centres and family medicine groups in Quebec	167
Box 9.5	Supporting cancer patients in Ontario	173

List of abbreviations

ABHI	Australian Better Health Initiative
ABS	Australian Bureau of Statistics
AHMAC	Australian Health Ministers Advisory Council
AHMC	Australian Health Ministers Conference
AIHW	Australian Institute of Health and Welfare
ALD	Affection de longue durée (long-term disease)
AMC	Associate medical centre (Quebec, Canada)
ANAES	French National Agency for Evaluation and Accreditation in Health
APCC	Australian Primary Care Collaboratives
APNA	Australian Practice Nursing Association
ARH	Agences régionales d'hospitalisation (regional authorities) (France)
AWBZ	Exceptional Medical Expenses Act (Netherlands)
AZM	Academic Hospital Maastricht
BiG	Law on Professionals in Health Care (Netherlands)
BMI	Body mass index
CALD	Culturally and linguistically diverse
CBO	Dutch Institute for Health Care Improvement
CCDPC	Centre for Chronic Disease Prevention and Control (Canada)
CCM	Chronic Care Model
CCO	Cancer Care Ontario
CDPM	Chronic Disease Prevention and Management (Canada)
CDSMP	Chronic Disease Self-Management Programme
CHSLD	Residential and long-term care centre (Quebec, Canada)
CLSC	Local community health centre (Quebec, Canada)
CMU	Universal Health Coverage Act (France)
COAG	Council of Australian Governments
COPD	Chronic obstructive pulmonary disease

CPOE	Computerized Physician Order Entry (Canada)
CQSI	Cancer Quality System Index (Canada)
CSSS	Health and social services centres (Canada)
CT	Computed tomography
DIEP	Diabetes Interactive Education Programme (Netherlands)
DMP	Disease management programme
DNDR	National Fund for the Development of Networks (France)
DRDR	Regional Fund for the Development of Networks (France)
EPC	Enhanced Primary Care (Australia)
EU	European Union
FAQVS	Fund for the Quality Improvement of Ambulatory Care (France)
FCC	Federation of Swedish County Councils
FHT	Family Health Team (Ontario, Canada)
FIQCS	Quality and Coordination of Care Fund (France)
FMG	Family medicine group (Quebec, Canada)
GBA	Federal Joint Committee (Germany)
GP	General practitioner
GPMP	General Practitioner Management Plan (Australia)
GPwSI	GPs with special interests
HAS	French National Authority for Health
HIV	Human immunodeficiency virus
IGAS	Audit Group of Health and Social Affairs (France)
IGZ	Dutch Health Care Inspectorate
ISIP	Integrated Service Improvement Programme (England)
IT	Information technology
KV	Regional physicians' associations (Germany)
LHIN	Local Health Integration Network (Ontario, Canada)
MAHS	More Allied Health Services (Australia)
MBS	Medicare Benefits Schedule (Australia)
MOBG	Ministry of Health steering committee (Netherlands)
MRI	Magnetic resonance imaging
NBHW	National Board of Health and Welfare (Sweden)
NCCZ	National Commission for the Chronically Ill (Netherlands)
NCDS	National Chronic Disease Strategy (Australia)

NDSS	National Diabetes Surveillance System (Canada)
NHG	Dutch College of General Practitioners
NHG-CAHAG	NHG Asthma and COPD GPs consulting group (Netherlands)
NHS	National Health Service (England)
NHMRC	National Health and Medical Research Council (Australia)
NHS	National Health Service
NICE	National Institute for Health and Clinical Excellence (England)
NIDP	National Integrated Diabetes Programme (Australia)
NIP	National Indicator Project (Denmark)
NIVEL	Netherlands Institute for Health Services Research
NPCC	National Primary Care Collaborative (Australia)
NPCG	National Panel for Chronically Ill People and Handicapped Persons (Netherlands)
NQPS	National Quality and Performance System (Australia)
NSF	National Service Framework (England)
NSW	New South Wales (Australia)
NVALT	Dutch Society of Doctors for Lung Diseases and Tuberculosis
NVAO	Accreditation Organisation of the Netherlands and Flanders
NzA	Dutch Health Care Authority
OCR	Ontario Cancer Registry (Ontario, Canada)
OECD	Organisation for Economic Co-operation and Development
PARR	Patients At Risk of Re-hospitalization (England)
PBS	Pharmaceutical Benefits Scheme (Australia)
PCT	Primary Care Trust (England)
PDA	Personal digital assistant
PHCC	Primary health care centre (Sweden)
PIMS	Pathology Information Management System (Canada)
PIN	Personal identification number
PIP	Practice Incentives Program (Australia)
POPP	Partnership for Older People Project (England)
PQVMC	Public Health Plan on Quality of Life for the Chronically Ill (France)

PRISMA	Program of Research to Integrate the Services for the Maintenance of Autonomy (Canada)
PRIISME	Programme to Integrate Information Services and Manage Education (Canada)
QOF	Quality and Outcomes Framework (England)
RHA	Regional Health Authority (Canada)
RIVM	National Institute for Public Health and the Environment (Netherlands)
RSA	Risk Structure Compensation Scheme (Germany)
RSAV	Regulation on Risk Structure Compensation (Germany)
RVP	Regional Vice-President
SALA	Swedish Association of Local Authorities
SALAR	Swedish Association of Local Authorities and Regions
SGB V	Social Code Book V (Germany)
SHA	Strategic Health Authority (England)
SHI	Social Health Insurance
SIKS	The integrated effort for people living with chronic diseases (project) (Denmark)
SIP	Service Incentive Payment (Australia)
SIPA	System of Integrated Services for the Frail Elderly (Canada)
SROS	Regional Strategic Health Plan (France)
SSFA	Social Security Funding Act (France)
SVR	Advisory Council on the Assessment of Developments in the Health Care System (Germany)
TCA	Team Care Arrangement (Australia)
URCAM	Regional Unions of Insurance Funds (France)
WGBO	Law on Medical Treatment by Professionals (Netherlands)
WGV	Law on the Prescription of Medicines (Netherlands)
WHIC	Western Health Information Collaborative (Canada)
WHO	World Health Organization
WMO	Social Support Act (Netherlands)

Foreword

The European Observatory is known for putting a spotlight on the challenge of chronic disease, a challenge which is placing such a heavy burden on health and social care systems in Europe and blighting the lives of millions of European citizens.

Through the inclusion in this study of the non-European countries of Australia and Canada, and the use of a SWOT (Strengths, Weaknesses, Opportunities and Threats) analysis, they have brought out 'lessons learned' and showed some best practice.

Comparisons are also skilfully demonstrated by describing a fictitious patient journey in each country, mostly using a 54-year-old woman with type 2 diabetes, COPD, a leg ulcer and moderate retinopathy, who is also slightly overweight, unemployed and lives alone. Diabetes is often the focus of many changes in disease management.

All the European countries studied have developed new approaches, but the most interesting seem to be relatively untried, as in England and Denmark, or affecting so few people, as in France, or with good uptake but little evaluation of any changes, as in Germany. The Netherlands has some good multidisciplinary approaches with a sound understanding of some of the professional barriers, whereas the new system developed by its neighbour Germany is dominated by doctors. The Swedish approach I found the most interesting: it is largely led by nurses, it is optimistic and yet it is honest.

Those patients with complex and difficult chronic disease are expected to navigate a health care system of equal complexity and the acronyms in many countries were so awful that I am amazed patients have any idea what is going on, let alone how to shape and influence their care.

This book brings together the approaches adopted by eight countries to address the policy issues necessary to provide high-quality and affordable health and social care for people suffering from chronic disease. It is an interesting book to read and the main authors have done a good job in pulling together all the different ideas and plans. For any country facing an unprecedented burden on its health care system, it will be important to recognize the seriousness of the current and future problems and to use new ways of working with all stakeholders to find solutions. Patients and their families need to be partners rather than passive recipients; all staff, not just doctors, need to be viewed as part of the solution and encouraged to innovate and search for better ways of delivering appropriate care.

Many of these diseases and their painful complications could have been prevented by earlier measures to prevent obesity and to encourage smoking cessation; the "lessons learned" need to be present in more than new care pathways but also expressed in ways to prevent many of these crippling diseases.

Christine Hancock
Oxford Health Alliance
October 2008

Acknowledgements

This volume is one of a series of books produced by the European Observatory on Health Systems and Policies. We are grateful to all the authors for their hard work, continuous support and enthusiasm in this project, as well as to Christine Hancock for contributing the Foreword.

In addition to the work of the authors, this work draws on a related volume edited by Ellen Nolte and Martin McKee. The contributors to that volume, including the editors, were Reinhard Busse, Elisabeth Chan, Anna Dixon, Carl-Ardy Dubois, Isabelle Durand-Zaleski, Daragh K Fahey, Nicholas Glasgow, Monique Hejmans, Izzat Jiwani, Martyn Jones, Cécile Knai, Nicholas Mays, Martin McKee, Ellen Nolte, Thomas E Novotny, Joceline Pomerleau, Mieke Rijken, Dhigna Rubiano, Debbie Singh and Marc Suhrcke.

We gratefully acknowledge the contributions of those who participated in a workshop held in London to discuss individual draft chapters of the volume. These were, in addition to the country study writers and the chapter authors, Allessandra Badellin, Armin Fidler, Bernard Merkel, Carmel Martin, Chris Ham, Christian Lüthje, Christine Hancock, Clare Siddall, Jill Farrington, Kenneth Thorpe, Kevin McCarthy, Margot Felix, Richard Saltman, Tit Albreht, Johan Calltorp and Ian Basnett. The workshop discussions provided an invaluable source for guiding this work further.

We are especially grateful to the National Institute for Health Research (NIHR) for their award of a Career Scientist Award to Dr Nolte without which this work would not have been possible.

We also gratefully acknowledge the time taken by the final reviewers of this volume, Christine Hancock and Colin J Kenny. We greatly benefited from their very helpful comments and suggestions.

Finally, this book would not have appeared without the able and patient support throughout the project of our colleagues in the Observatory. In particular, we would like to thank Caroline White and Sue Gammerman, who, with the invaluable assistance of Maria Teresa Marchetti, Pieter Herroelen and Alain Cochez, managed all administrative matters related to this work, and organized the workshop in London. We are also very grateful to Jonathan North for managing the production process, and to Nicole Satterly for copy-editing the manuscript.

List of contributors

Carl-Ardy Dubois is Associate Professor in the Faculty of Nursing Sciences at the University of Montreal.

Isabelle Durand-Zaleski is Professor of Medicine at the University of Paris and head of the Public Health Department at Henri Mondor hospital, Paris, France.

Daragh K Fahey is a public health consultant who is Director of Service Development for UnitedHealth.

Anne Frølich, is Senior Consultant at the Clinical Unit of Health Promotion at Bispebjerg Hospital, and external Lecturer at the Institute of Public Health, University of Copenhagen.

Nicholas Glasgow was the Foundation Director of the Australian Primary Health Care Research Institute and is Dean of Medicine and Health Sciences in the College of Medicine Biology and Environment at the Australian National University.

Mark Harris is Professor of General Practice and Executive Director of the Centre for Primary Health Care and Equity, University of New South Wales, Sydney, Australia.

Iqbal Hasan is a project officer at the Centre for Primary Health Care and Equity, School of Public Health and Community Medicine, University of New South Wales, Australia.

Izzat Jiwani is a research associate to the Chair of Governance and Transformation of Health Organizations at the University of Montreal, and has an independent practice as a health policy researcher and management consultant.

Tanisha Jowsey is a Research Officer at the Australian Primary Health Care Research Institute at the Australian National University.

Ingvar Karlberg is Professor of Public Health and Health Systems Research at Göteborg University and Medical Advisor to the Regional Authority Västra Götaland, Sweden.

Eveline Klein Lankhorst is a Doctoral Research Student and Research Assistant at the Health Services Research Unit, London School of Hygiene & Tropical Medicine.

Cécile Knai is a Research Fellow at the London School of Hygiene & Tropical Medicine.

Allan Krasnik is Professor of Social Medicine at the Department of Health Services Research at the Institute of Public Health, University of Copenhagen, and Director of the Master of Public Health programme at the University of Copenhagen.

Martin McKee is Head of Research Policy of the European Observatory on Health Systems and Policies and Professor of European Public Health at the London School of Hygiene & Tropical Medicine.

Ellen Nolte is a Senior Lecturer at the London School of Hygiene & Tropical Medicine and Honorary Senior Research Fellow at the European Observatory on Health Systems and Policies.

Olivier Obrecht, specialized in public health. He was in charge of developing guidelines for the management of the care of persons with chronic conditions at the Haute Autorité de Santé, France.

Michaela Schiøtz is a Doctoral Research Student in Public Health at the Institute of Public Health, University of Copenhagen, and Visiting Research Scholar at LSE Health, London School of Economics and Political Science.

Ulrich Siering is Deputy Head of the Quality of Health Care Department at the Institute for Quality and Efficiency in Health Care (IQWiG), Germany.

Debra de Silva is Head of Evaluation at The Evidence Centre, providing independent research, public consultations and evidence reviews for health and social service organizations throughout the world. She is also Senior Associate at the University of Birmingham.

Cor Spreeuwenberg is a retired Professor in Integrated Chronic Care at the Research School Caphri, Maastricht University Center of Medicine (MUMC); he is still active in promoting the practical development and scientific evaluation of innovative integrated care programmmes for people with chronic conditions in the Netherlands and Europe.

Nicholas Zwar is Professor of General Practice in the School of Public Health and Community Medicine, University of New South Wales, Sydney, Australia.

Chapter 1
Managing chronic conditions: An introduction to the experience in eight countries

Ellen Nolte, Martin McKee, Cécile Knai

Introduction

While only a few things can be predicted with certainty, one thing that seems certain is that the future of health care will be dominated by the challenge of complex chronic disorders. The 20th century witnessed an epidemiological transition in which the conquest of many epidemic infectious diseases was counterbalanced by a steady rise in chronic noncommunicable conditions, many associated with important changes in lifestyle (Omran 1971). Many of these conditions are a consequence of accumulated exposure to chronic disease risk factors over a person's lifetime (Ben-Shlomo & Kuh 2002, Janssen & Kunst 2005); modern medicine may be able to control them, but not cure them. With a growing body of research identifying factors associated with healthy ageing (Depp, Glatt & Jeste 2007), and although the onset of these conditions can be postponed as populations become older, due to a combination of longer survival and falling birth rates, the share of the population living with these conditions will inevitably increase. Thus, in the countries of the European Union (EU), in 2006, between one fifth and over 40% of the population aged 15 years and over reported a long-standing health problem (TNS Opinion & Social 2007). Importantly, there will be a growing number of people with multiple health problems, most common among older people, with an estimated two thirds of those who have reached pensionable age having at least two chronic conditions

(Deutsches Zentrum für Altersfragen 2005, Van den Akker et al. 1998, Wolff, Starfield & Anderson 2002).

Indeed, it is the co-existence of multiple disorders that poses the greatest challenges. Thus, it is not unusual for an 80-year-old person to suffer from five or six conditions, controlled by as many potentially interacting pharmaceuticals the metabolism of which is affected by an ageing body. This is not a problem that lends itself to simple responses. Instead, chronic diseases require a complex response, over a prolonged time period, coordinating inputs from a wide range of health professionals, essential medicines and – where appropriate – monitoring equipment, all of which is optimally embedded within a system that promotes patient empowerment.

With many health systems still largely built around an acute, episodic model of care, the challenge facing health policy-makers today is how to put in place a response that better meets the needs of people with complex chronic health problems. As health systems differ widely, each must find their own solution. Even within superficially similar systems there may be marked differences in professional roles, in coordination mechanisms and in care settings. Nonetheless, there is scope to learn from others; a process that has already begun. In this book we seek to facilitate this process, by drawing together a series of studies describing how selected countries have responded to these common challenges. This book should be read in association with a thematic analysis, published in collaboration with the European Observatory on Health Systems and Policies, that draws on these country studies and a wider range of literature to explore how health systems can respond to the needs of people with chronic conditions (Nolte & McKee 2008a).

Scope

In response to the emerging challenge posed by chronic diseases, many countries have experimented with new models of, or approaches to, health care delivery designed to achieve better coordination of services across the continuum of care required by people with chronic illnesses. A recent review of organizational innovations in a range of European countries illustrated considerable variation in the approaches to chronic disease management that are being implemented in different health care settings (McKee & Nolte 2004). It found that the characteristics of each health system were important determinants of success in introducing new patterns of service delivery. It suggests, for example, that tax-based systems seem to find it easier to implement organizational innovations that involve coordination across interfaces, while social insurance systems seem to face major difficulties in implementing coordinated approaches to care due to their tendency to have a strict separation between ambulatory and inpatient care sectors. However, many of the conclusions of the review were tentative, reflecting the scarcity of robust evaluations that go beyond comparisons of individual interventions to take a broad perspective on how each health system addresses the needs of patients with chronic health problems.

In this volume we build on the earlier review, providing an in-depth assessment of how health systems in eight countries have responded to the rising burden of chronic disease. Given the marked lack of information in many places, the choice of countries is to some extent pragmatic. Although the main criterion has been to include a mix of systems with different approaches to funding and delivering health care, an important consideration was the ability to identify authors who had in-depth knowledge of the country in question and could assemble the appropriate information. In the future, it will hopefully be possible to take a more systematic approach. For example, one might compile data on outcomes of chronic disease, from which countries could be drawn to include high, medium and low performers. Unfortunately, as we have shown elsewhere (Pomerleau, Knai & Nolte 2008), with the exception of mortality (McKee & Nolte 2004), there are very few comparable data available at the time of writing that would allow for such a systematic selection process.

The countries included are Denmark, England, France, Germany, the Netherlands and Sweden, with the addition of Australia and Canada, which, while outside the European region can nevertheless provide important and useful lessons for the care of patients with chronic conditions in Europe.

A few words of explanation are necessary. Although the United Kingdom is, politically, a single country, the health systems in its constituent parts are increasingly divergent. We have therefore focused on the situation in England, which has been the setting for a large number of initiatives. Some may also question the exclusion of the United States, often seen as the origin of much health care innovation. However, the United States is an outlier among industrialized countries, most obviously in its failure to achieve universal coverage but also in the sheer complexity of its health care system and, although less-well recognized, in its very much worse outcomes for chronic disease compared to those in Europe, as expressed in terms of mortality rates that are typically about five times higher (McKee & Nolte 2004). Still, many of the models of care being adopted in Europe have originated in the United States, as illustrated in the following chapters.

The overall aim that we set ourselves in this book was to compile an in-depth assessment of the health system response to the rising burden of chronic disease in each of the eight countries, by focusing on three key areas: (1) a detailed examination of the current situation; (2) a description of the policy framework and future scenarios; and (3) evaluation and lessons learnt, building on a common template developed by the editors. The template was informed, to great extent, by the Chronic Care Model (CCM) developed by Wagner and colleagues in Seattle (Wagner, Austin & Von Korff 1996). This model presents a structure for organizing health care; it comprises four interacting components that are considered key to providing high-quality care for those with chronic health problems: self-management support, delivery system design, decision support, and clinical information systems. These are set within a health system context that links an appropriately organized delivery system with complementary community resources and policies. Following this structure, the country assessments presented here therefore provide (1) a summary of the key features of the country's health system; (2) an overview of services provided for patients with chronic disease, describing types and delivery models in place, providers involved, key strategies adopted to manage chronic disease, distribution of related services and population covered; (3) an assessment of key health system features supporting the development or implementation of delivery models or programmes, including the use of targets, standards and guidelines, health care workforce development and evaluation and lessons learnt; and (4) future prospects, including an analysis of the strengths and weaknesses of approaches and strategies in place.

It is important to note that, although the country assessments were based on a common template, the way in which they are described varies. For example, the Canadian analysis has a provincial focus, reflecting the highly decentralized nature of Canadian health care, with a wide range of strategies and initiatives being adopted by individual provinces. A comprehensive analysis of all the initiatives that exist across Canada would have gone far beyond the scope of this book. The authors chose to concentrate on the province of Ontario, drawing on the example of cancer care. Although not always thought of as a "chronic disease", the advent of new treatments mean that many people who would once have died from cancer are now living with it, in many cases changing it from a rapidly progressive fatal disease to a chronic conditon. The analysis of Cancer Care Ontario (CCO) illustrates how a (regional) health system has transformed the provision of care, bringing together a once fragmented aglomeration of care providers into an integrated system that is able to address the changing needs of cancer patients. Similarly, although the template asked for a description of a typical pathway for a patient with defined characteristics, this was not always possible because of the absence of a pathway that was "typical".

It is also important to recognize what this book is not. It does not seek to appraise systematically the findings from each of the eight countries. Instead, a detailed assessment can be found in an accompanying volume, which was informed extensively by the material included here (Nolte & McKee 2008a, Nolte &

McKee 2008b). Drawing in part on that detailed assessment, the following section briefly reviews some of the main observations that have emerged from the experiences of the countries described in subsequent chapters. We hope that this will contribute to an agenda for future work on these issues.

Experience in eight countries: key observations

The chapters in this book show that there are many different strategies being implemented to address chronic disease in the countries reviewed, with different systems at different stages of the process and with different degrees of comprehensiveness. Perhaps not surprisingly, the approaches adopted often reflect the characteristics of each health system, in terms of their governance mechanisms and the relationships between, and responsibilities of, different stakeholders in the regulation, funding and delivery of health care. However, some common features do seem to be emerging.

Given the richness of the material presented in this volume, in this introduction we focus on a few selected observations, concentrating on core features of health care organization and financing and how these tend to facilitate, or hinder, the implementation of structured approaches to chronic disease management.

In countries where primary care is based largely on multi-professional teams of physicians, nurses and other health professionals and where patients are registered with a specific primary care facility, there has been a progressive increase in the role of nurses in managing many chronic diseases. This commonly takes the form of nurse-led clinics, discharge planning and/or case management. This has been the case in Sweden and England and, more recently, the Netherlands. Thus, in **Sweden** nurse-led clinics are now common at primary health care centres (PHCC) and in hospital polyclinics, managing diabetes and hypertension, with some also managing allergy/asthma/chronic obstructive pulmonary disease (COPD), psychiatric disorders and heart failure. By the late 1990s, two thirds of hospitals had established nurse-led heart failure clinics, with nurses empowered to change medication regimes within agreed protocols (Stromberg et al. 2001). There is now considerable evidence from various countries and for different diseases that this approach yields better results than traditional physician-led care, and may also reduce costs (Singh 2005, Vrijhoef et al. 2001), although given differences in professional roles within Europe, some caution may be required in applying this model elsewhere (Smith et al. 2001).

In **England**, there is considerable local diversity in the response to chronic diseases, but common elements include nurse-led clinics and other nurse-led services, including specialist nurses as case managers of individuals with complex needs ("community matrons"), and multidisciplinary teams. Community matrons are central to the Government's approach to supporting patients with chronic conditions. The 2004 National Health Service (NHS) Improvement Plan stipulated the introduction of case management in all Primary Care Trusts (PCTs), which are responsible for purchasing health services in England. Case management was to be delivered by over 3000 community matrons to be appointed to support approximately 250 000 patients with complex chronic conditions (Department of Health 2004). The anticipated benefits included improved quality of care and, by preventing or delaying complications, reduced (emergency) admissions and long hospital stays, although initial evidence from pilots casts some doubt on whether this can be achieved. A focus on chronic disease is also apparent in the system now in place to pay general practitioners (GPs), which explicitly rewards quality of care and health outcomes. This has been facilitated by the high level of computerization in English general practices.

In the **Netherlands**, nurses have been playing an increasingly important role in arrangements for what is termed "transmural care", which since the early 1990s has sought to bridge the divide between secondary care and alternative settings for those who are not able to return to a fully independent life (Van der Linden, Spreeuwenberg & Schrijvers 2001). Transmural care arrangements have frequently involved specialized nurses, who have been trained in the care of patients with specific chronic conditions, and discharge liaison nurses. More recently, there has been a move towards disease management models, with nurse-led clinics at their core, as in Maastricht (Vrijhoef et al. 2001).

In contrast, in countries such as **Germany**, which offers patients free choice of both family practitioners and specialists working in ambulatory care, physicians are more likely to work as individual practitioners, with, until recently, a strict separation between the ambulatory and hospital sector. As a consequence, the German response has tended to follow the United States' approach by introducing structured disease management programmes (DMPs) for selected conditions. Recognizing the limited ability of the system to support patients with complex needs, from 1993 the Government successively introduced provisions to enable the development of more coordinated models of care. In 2002 the Government formally introduced DMPs as a means to improve the quality of care for those with chronic illness (Busse 2004).

DMPs are provided in addition to existing health services. As such, they have not fundamentally altered the existing structure of primary care in Germany. However, in the 2004 Social Health Insurance Modernization Act, the German Government also established mechanisms to facilitate coordination between the ambulatory and hospital sectors by removing certain legal and financial obstacles. This has enabled health insurance funds to designate financial resources for selective contracting with individual providers or networks of providers (Busse and Riesberg 2004).

As in Germany, there has been concern in the **French** health care system about the lack of coordination and continuity of care, both at the ambulatory level as well as at the interface between ambulatory and hospital care (Sandier, Paris & Polton 2004). This slowly changed following the 1996 Juppé reforms that introduced mechanisms designed to stimulate experiments with different provider networks at local level. Initiatives were eventually formalized under the 2002 legislation on patients' rights and quality of care, which brought together all initiatives under a single "health networks" (Réseaux de Santé) umbrella, aiming to strengthen the coordination, continuity and interdisciplinarity of health care provision, with a particular focus on selected population groups, disorders or activities (Frossard et al. 2002). Subsequently, the 2004 Public Health Law defined a series of health targets for (chronic) diseases and risk factors, followed by the 2007 national public health plan for people with chronic illness (Ministère de la Santé et des Solidarités 2007). At the same time, the 2004 Health Insurance Law reformed the traditional long-term disease (ALD, affections de longue durée) procedure, which exempts patients with long-term conditions from co-payments if their care adheres to evidence-based guidelines. Although individually viewed as positive developments, it has been argued that these initiatives lack an integrative vision, with no clearly defined objectives, procedures for implementation, or incentives and sanctions. There is an expectation that the 2007 national plan will provide an important step towards a more coherent approach to chronic disease.

In **Canada**, individual provinces have responsibility for health service organization, within a national framework of entitlements. While there is no single unified vision of coordinated care, efforts are under way across the country to improve coordination and continuity of care through shared governance of a broad range of health services and increased collaboration among health providers. Notable examples can be found in Ontario, Quebec, Alberta and British Columbia. For example, Ontario introduced local Family Health Teams (FHTs) (Southeastern Ontario District Health Council 2004), which aim to enhance access to and coordination of care while encouraging and facilitating multidisciplinary service provision (Ontario Ministry of Health and Long-Term Care 2001, Tuohy 2002). This strategy has been complemented by the more recently established Local Health Integration Networks (LHINs), created in 2005. These are local governance structures with a mandate to plan, coordinate and fund local health services within specified geographic areas. Many have identified chronic disease prevention and management as a priority. In Quebec, initiatives to enhance chronic care have been embedded in an overall strategy to improve health and social care within the scope of the available resources. This has involved the creation of local services networks (health and social services centres, CSSS) which bring together all care providers in a region to develop partnerships between relevant groups (such as physicians and community organizations). These are tasked with ensuring provision of a comprehensive package of services stretching from prevention to end-of-life care.

Like Canada, a key feature of the **Danish** health system is its high level of decentralization, in which regions and municipalities are largely responsible for organizing health care. However, in 2002, Denmark did develop a national vision of chronic disease control (Danish Ministry of the Interior and Health 2003), with a 2006 report setting out options for improving care coordination for those with chronic conditions (Danish National Board of Health 2006). Many of the options proposed are in the form of general recommendations, although some are more specific, with a major focus on structured approaches to supporting patient self-management and disease management. At the same time, municipal health centres are being established and evaluated, primarily targeting elderly people and those with chronic health problems.

What these last four countries have in common is a tradition whereby primary care has been provided by doctors, typically in single-handed practices with few support staff. These countries have found it challenging to develop and implement new roles and competencies. This is in part because of payment modalities, as shown in the chapters that follow, as well as legal provisions, such as in France, where redefining roles and delegating tasks to nonmedical personnel requires changes in the law on professional responsibilities. In addition, in countries where nurses have traditionally played a minimal role in primary care, as in Canada (Bailey, Jones & Way 2006), Germany (Rosemann et al. 2006) and Australia (Oldroyd et al. 2003), there are often professional concerns among physicians about delegating tasks.

Several countries have introduced financial incentives for providers and/or purchasers/payers to strengthen care coordination or implement structured DMPs. Examples include Australia, Denmark, England, France and Germany. Thus, the **Australian** Commonwealth Government introduced an Enhanced Primary Care (EPC) scheme in 1999 as a means to improve coordination of care for people with chronic conditions and complex care needs (Healy, Sharman & Lokuga 2006). The scheme provides a framework for a multidisciplinary approach to health care, which, along with the Service Incentive Payments (SIP) and Practice Incentives Program (PIP), offers financial incentives to

GPs to encourage coordination of care for patients with chronic conditions. Uptake of these initiatives by GPs has, however, been variable, which has been attributed largely to administrative complexity and inflexible structures that impede the implementation of structured multidisciplinary care in general practice (Oldroyd et al. 2003, Zwar et al. 2005). An amended EPC scheme came into effect in July 2005, offering additional options for managing patients with chronic conditions and complex needs in general practice (Newland & Zwar 2006). However, it remains uncertain whether the revised system will overcome the difficulties observed previously.

The **German** DMPs are funded by means of a change in the Risk Structure Compensation Scheme (RSA), which creates strong incentives for sickness funds to enrol patients. They may also provide considerable financial incentives for physicians participating in the scheme. Preliminary evidence indicates some success in terms of uptake and patient outcomes (Nordrheinische Gemeinsame Einrichtung Disease-Management-Programme GbR 2005, Petro et al. 2005), with more recent evaluations pointing to improvements in the quality of care provided to patients (Szecsenyi et al. 2008, Gapp et al. 2008). However, although DMPs are now an integral component of the German health care sector, their effectiveness and financial linkages to the RSA continue to be debated (Gerst & Korzilius 2005).

As noted above, in **England**, strategies to improve the care for those with chronic conditions in primary care have been supported by a new system of paying for primary care, based on a complex Quality and Outcomes Framework (QOF) introduced in 2004, and with data published annually. The QOF is designed to provide appropriate financial incentives to encourage general practices to provide ongoing high-quality management of 10 chronic conditions including diabetes, hypertension and asthma (Roland 2004). By September 2005 almost all general practices in England had joined the QOF scheme, achieving, on average, 91% of the maximum achievable score, indicating considerable progress in quality of care for patients with chronic conditions such as diabetes and heart disease (Cole 2005). However, variation in the quality of care provided in general practices has persisted (Campbell et al. 2005) and there has been concern about the quality of care for patients with conditions not covered under the QOF (Wilson, Buck & Ham 2005), although revision of the Framework has been undertaken to account for "wider health and well-being outcomes" by 2008–2009 (Department of Health 2006).

Other approaches to incentivize coordination among providers also involve changes to funding mechanisms. For example, the recent structural reforms in **Denmark** that ascribed municipalities a greater role in health mean that the municipalities are now required to contribute 20% of total health care funding. This was designed to encourage municipalities to invest in health promotion and preventive treatment, while developing alternatives to hospital services (Ankjaer-Jensen & Christiansen 2007). However, there are concerns that this could impede coordination and may potentially lead to a duplication of services provided by municipalities and regions.

An important observation is how payment systems can often hinder the delegation of tasks from doctors to other health professionals. For example, in Australia, although the EPC scheme was intended to encourage multidisciplinary care, its impact has been limited because payment for participation in many activities has been limited to GPs. A lack of appropriate incentives has also been identified as creating barriers to greater involvement by GPs in integrated approaches to care in Denmark and the Netherlands. In France, the payment of providers on a fee-for-service basis does not encourage improved coordination between physicians and nurses. As Busse & Mays (2008) note, those health systems with a tradition of patient choice of any provider, little or no enrolment with particular providers and/or of paying for services episodically using fee-for-service payments as the predominant method of reimbursement seem to face the greatest challenges in adapting their payment arrangements to provide effective chronic care. Such systems tend to discourage continuity of care or a population perspective. In contrast, systems with strong primary health care are more likely to give greater attention to the management of people with chronic conditions and to obtain better results.

The chapters that follow examine the experiences of these eight countries in more detail.

References

Ankjaer-Jensen A, Christiansen T (2007). Municipal co-payment for health care services. *Health Policy Monitor*, 10 (October) (http://www.hpm.org/survey/dk/a10/3, accessed 11 February 2008).

Bailey P, Jones L, Way D (2006). Family physician/nurse practitioner: stories of collaboration. *Journal of Advanced Nursing*, 53(4):381–391.

Ben-Shlomo Y, Kuh D (2002). A life course approach to chronic disease epidemiology: conceptual models, empirical challenges, and interdisciplinary perspectives. *International Journal of Epidemiology*, 31:285–293.

Busse R (2004). Disease management programmes in Germany's statutory health insurance system. *Health Affairs*, 23:56–67.

Busse R, Mays N (2008). Paying for chronic disease care. In: Nolte E, McKee M (eds). *Caring for people with chronic conditions: a health system perspective.* Maidenhead, Open University Press:195–221.

Busse R, Riesberg A (2004). Health care systems in transition: Germany. *Health Systems in Transition*, 6(9):1–234.

Campbell S et al. (2005). Improvements in quality of clinical care in English general practice 1998–2003: longitudinal observational study. *British Medical Journal*, 331:1121–1125.

Cole A (2005). UK GP activity exceeds expectations. *British Medical Journal*, 331:536.

Danish Ministry of the Interior and Health (2003). *Healthy throughout life – the targets and strategies for public health policy of the Government of Denmark, 2002–2010.* Copenhagen, Danish Ministry of the Interior and Health.

Danish National Board of Health (2006). *Chronic conditions – Patients, healthcare and community.* Copenhagen, Danish National Board of Health.

Department of Health (2004). *The NHS Improvement Plan.* London, Department of Health.

Department of Health (2006). *Our health, our care, our say: a new direction for community services.* London, The Stationery Office.

Depp CA, Glatt SJ, Jeste DV (2007). Recent advances in research on successful or healthy ageing. *Current Psychiatry Reports*, 9(1):7–13.

Deutsches Zentrum für Altersfragen (2005). *Gesundheit und Gesundheitsversorgung. Der Alterssurvey: Aktuelles auf einen Blick, ausgewählte Ergebnisse.* Bonn, Bundesministeriums für Familie, Senioren, Frauen und Jugend (http://www.dza.de/download/Gesundheit.pdf, accessed 12 December 2006).

Frossard M et al. (2002). *Providing integrated health and social care for older persons in France – An old idea with a great future.* Paris, Union nationale interfédérale des oeuvres et organismes privés sanitaires et sociaux.

Gapp O et al. (2008). Disease management programmes for patients with coronary heart disease. An empirical study of German programmes. *Health Policy* (In press).

Gerst T, Korzilius H (2005). Disease-Management-Programme: Viel Geld im Spiel. *Deutsches Ärzteblatt*, 102:A2904–9.

Healy J, Sharman E, Lokuga B (2006). Australia: Health system review. *Health Systems in Transition*, 8(5):1–158.

Janssen F, Kunst A (2005). Cohort patterns in mortality trends among the elderly in seven European countries, 1950–1999. *International Journal of Epidemiology*, 34:1149–1159.

McKee M, Nolte E (2004). Responding to the challenge of chronic diseases: ideas from Europe. *Clinical Medicine*, 4:336–342.

Ministère de la Santé et des Solidarités (2007). *Plan pour l'amélioration de la qualité de vie des personnes atteintes de maladies chroniques*. Paris, Ministère de la Santé et des Solidarités.

Newland J, Zwar N (2006). General practice and the management of chronic conditions – where to now? *Australian Family Physician*, 35(1–2):16–19.

Nolte E, McKee M (eds) (2008a). *Caring for people with chronic conditions: a health system perspective*. Maidenhead, Open University Press.

Nolte E, McKee M (2008b). Making it happen. In: Nolte E, McKee M (eds). *Caring for people with chronic conditions: A health system perspective*. Maidenhead, Open University Press:222–224.

Nordrheinische Gemeinsame Einrichtung Disease-Management-Programme GbR (2005). *Qualitätssicherungsbericht 2004 Disease-Management-Programme in Nordrhein*. Düsseldorf, Nordrheinische Gemeinsame Einrichtung Disease-Management-Programme GbR.

Oldroyd J et al. (2003). Providing health care for people with chronic illness: the views of Australian GPs. *Medical Journal of Australia*, 179(1):30–33.

Omran AR (1971). The epidemiologic transition. A theory of the epidemiology of population change. *Milbank Memorial Fund Quarterly*, 49(4):509–538.

Ontario Ministry of Health and Long-Term Care (2001). *Evaluation of primary care reform in Ontario. Phase 2 interim report*. Toronto, ON, Ontario Ministry of Health and Long-Term Care, PriceWaterhouseCoopers.

Petro W et al. (2005). Effizienz eines Disease Management Programmes bei Asthma. *Pneumologie*, 59:101–107.

Pomerleau J, Knai C, Nolte E (2008). The burden of chronic disease in Europe. In: Nolte E, McKee M (eds). *Caring for people with chronic conditions: A health system perspective*. Maidenhead, Open University Press:15–42.

Roland M (2004). Linking physicians' pay to the quality of care – a major experiment in the United Kingdom. *New England Journal of Medicine*, 351:1448–1454.

Rosemann T et al. (2006). How can the practice nurse be more involved in the care of the chronically ill? The perspectives of GPs, patients and practice nurses. *BioMed Central Family Practice*, 7:14.

Sandier S, Paris V, Polton D (2004). Health systems in transition: France. *Health Systems in Transition*, 6(2):1–145.

Singh D (2005). *Which staff improve care for people with long-term conditions? A rapid review of the literature.* Birmingham, NHS Modernisation Agency and University of Birmingham.

Smith B et al. (2001). Home care by outreach nursing for chronic obstructive pulmonary disease. *Cochrane Database of Systematic Reviews*, (3):CD000994.

Southeastern Ontario District Health Council (2004). *Primary health care. Models and initiatives.* Kingston, ON, Southeastern Ontario District Health Council.

Stromberg A et al. (2001). Nurse-led heart failure clinics in Sweden. *European Journal of Heart Failure*, 3(1):139–144.

Szecsenyi J et al. (2008). German diabetes disease management programs are appropriate for restructuring care according to the chronic care model: an evaluation with the patient assessment of chronic illness care instrument. *Diabetes Care*, 31:1150–1154.

TNS Opinion & Social (2007). *Health in the European Union*. Special Eurobarometer 272e. Brussels, European Commission.

Van den Akker M et al. (1998). Multi-morbidity in general practice: prevalence, incidence, and determinants of co-occurring chronic and recurrent diseases. *Journal of Clinical Epidemiology*, 51:367–375.

Van der Linden BA, Spreeuwenberg C, Schrijvers JP (2001). Integration of care in the Netherlands: the development of transmural care since 1994. *Health Policy*, 55:111–120.

Vrijhoef et al. (2001). Adoption of disease management model for diabetes in region of Maastricht. *British Medical Journal*, 323:983–985.

Wagner E, Austin B, Von Korff M (1996). Organizing care for patients with chronic illness. *Milbank Quarterly*, 74:511–544.

Wilson T, Buck D, Ham C (2005). Rising to the challenge: will the NHS support people with long-term conditions? *British Medical Journal*, 330:657–661.

Wolff J, Starfield B, Anderson GF (2002). Prevalence, expenditures, and complications of multiple chronic conditions in the elderly, *Archives of Internal Medicine*, 162:2269–2276.

Zwar N et al. (2005). General practitioner views on barriers and facilitators to implementation of the Asthma 3+ Visit Plan. *Medical Journal of Australia*, 183:64–67.

Chapter 2
Denmark

Michaela Schiøtz, Anne Frølich, Allan Krasnik

Context

The Danish health care sector is predominantly public, financed mainly by local and national taxes, and in large part managed at regional level. The role of the central Government is almost exclusively to regulate, supervise and finance; the regions manage somatic and psychiatric health care services in public hospitals, as well as primary health services. The regions receive funding from the national Government and the municipalities. They own and run most hospitals and finance self-employed health professionals in independent practice, mainly on a fee-for-service basis. Reimbursement levels for private practitioners and salaries for employed health professionals are agreed through negotiations between the Danish Regions and the different professional associations. The regions are responsible for the development of overall strategies for prevention and treatment of chronic conditions, including disease management programmes.

The municipalities are responsible for care of the elderly, social psychiatry, prevention and health promotion, as well as rehabilitation where this is not a direct consequence of inpatient hospital care. Social services delivered by the municipalities include care of elderly people, disabled people and people with chronic diseases, including mental disorders, carried out in peoples' homes and in community mental health care centres (Strandberg-Larsen et al. 2007). The municipalities are responsible for rehabilitation of those with chronic conditions and for the establishment of a new delivery model: health care centres.

Access to hospitals and GPs is free of charge for all residents, although pharmaceuticals, dental care and some other services require co-payment.

General practice gatekeeping has been a key feature of the Danish system for many years (Strandberg-Larsen et al. 2007).

Recent health care reforms have been focusing increasingly on patient choice, reducing waiting times, quality assurance and coordination of care. A major structural reform in 2007 changed the political and administrative landscape dramatically, grouping the previous 14 counties into 5 newly established regions and reducing the number of municipalities from 275 to 98. At the same time, responsibility for prevention and rehabilitation was transferred from the regional to the municipal level (Strandberg-Larsen et al. 2007).

The distribution of responsibility between regions and municipalities in the health care sector is based on the principle that municipalities are responsible for home care and rehabilitation outside hospital, as well as for disease prevention and health promotion, with regions responsible for everything else. There is, however, concern that the structural reform might lead to unintended fragmentation of the system as it places considerable demands on those responsible for coordinating activities between the municipalities and the regions. A system of mandatory regional health care agreements was put in place, replacing the previous health plans, to strengthen the coherence between prevention, treatment and care. The health care agreements are expected to comply with centrally defined requirements, with joint service goals being published. They cover, for example, procedures for discharge of vulnerable and elderly patients, social services for people with mental disorders, and prevention and rehabilitation. The health care agreements are concluded by regional consultative committees, comprising representatives from regions, municipalities, and private practices. The committees act as arbitrator among the parties and the final agreements are published (Strandberg-Larsen et al. 2007).

Analysing the response

Approaches to chronic disease management

In 2002 the Danish Government released a major public health policy document, *Healthy throughout Life – the targets and strategies for public health policy of the Government of Denmark 2002–2010* (Ministry of the Interior and Health 2003). *Healthy throughout Life* places a special focus on efforts to reduce the major preventable diseases and disorders, looking in particular at type 2 diabetes, preventable cancers, cardiovascular diseases, osteoporosis, musculoskeletal disorders, hypersensitivity disorders (asthma and allergy), mental disorders and COPD.

As part of the Healthy throughout Life policy, the National Board of Health subsequently initiated a project on major preventable diseases and disorders, aiming to develop and strengthen systematic efforts to prevent the eight diseases and disease groups targeted by the Healthy throughout Life strategy and to contribute to integrating disease prevention and health promotion systematically within Denmark's health care system (National Board of Health 2004).

The National Board of Health project identified nine sub-projects that focus on (1) self-management; (2) promoting health and preventing disease in general practice; (3) national recommendations for the early detection of COPD and for pulmonary rehabilitation; (4) systematic comprehensive cardiac rehabilitation guidelines; (5) national recommendations to prevent falls and bone fractures among elderly people; (6) musculoskeletal disorders; (7) early detection and preventive treatment of hypersensitivity disorders; (8) physical activity in hospital; and (9) including data on physical inactivity and inadequate diet as risk factors for illness in patient records.

These sub-projects thus cover a range of activities along the continuum of care, stretching from prevention and early detection through to management of risk factors and rehabilitation, targeting a variety of chronic conditions as well as promoting patient education and intersectoral efforts involving the health care system. The primary roles of the National Board of Health in this project include facilitating, initiating, coordinating and providing documentation (National Board of Health 2004).

These efforts were followed, in 2005, by a report setting out options for improving care for those with chronic conditions (National Board of Health 2006). It builds, in part, on experience with initiatives at regional level that have been implemented during recent years. These include, among others, a patient self-management support programme based on the Chronic Disease Self-Management Programme (CDSMP) developed at Stanford University in the United States (Lorig 1993). There is also a fairly high number of disease-specific education classes offered to patients in the Danish health care system, targeting a range of conditions including diabetes, asthma, arthritis, osteoporosis and certain mental and neurological disorders. These have been implemented since the 1990s with the goal of reducing the number of avoidable hospitalizations and length of stay (Willaing, Folmann & Gisselbaek 2005).

From 2005 the central Government has partly supported the implementation of 18 health care centres throughout the country, investing a total of DDK 100 million (€13.4 million). A general model for the management of chronic disease is planned to be launched in the near future, based on the Chronic Care Model (CCM) developed in the United States (Bodenheimer, Wagner & Grumbach 2002). These developments are described in more detail later.

Distribution, uptake and coverage

There is currently no systematic disease-related registration or documentation of services delivered in the primary care sector. Several projects, such as the Danish Quality Improvement Project for General Practitioners, focus on the development of quality assessment systems but have not yet been implemented. There is some evidence that Danish health professionals spend between 0.5 and 2.5 hours a day advising patients on lifestyle changes (Nielsen et al. 2006). However, they only infrequently refer patients to other services that might help in this role, or use written materials to support lifestyle changes. One third of health personnel have reported receiving training on giving lifestyle advice within the preceding year.

The structural reform has led municipalities to carry out a number of new health care tasks, including rehabilitation, disease prevention and health promotion. Health care centres are currently being piloted, and are partly funded by the Government. These are viewed as possible organizational units to take on some of these new tasks. However, there is no common definition of what constitutes a health care centre and consequently the range of services provided by centres varies widely, from primary prevention to rehabilitation. The majority of centres focus on preventive and/or rehabilitative services for people with chronic conditions. The following section describes the Østerbro health care centre in Copenhagen municipality as an example of a health care centre that focuses on rehabilitation for people with chronic conditions.

Østerbro health care centre

Established in 2005, the Østerbro health care centre serves 82 000 of the over 600 000 residents in Copenhagen. It provides physiotherapy, dietary counselling, education, and smoking cessation courses to patients suffering from a range of conditions including heart disease, COPD, type 2 diabetes and balance problems following falls, as well as, more recently, ischaemic heart disease and metabolic syndrome, chosen because there is good evidence of the effectiveness of rehabilitation in this area.

The establishment of Østerbro health care centre was supported by Copenhagen municipality, funding a total of DDK 5 million (€670 000) for start-up and operating costs. The city's Health and Social Administration worked with the municipal hospital and GPs to create a local chronic care project. The project, entitled An Integrated Effort for People with Chronic Diseases (SIKS), aims to strengthen integrated care pathways and promote rehabilitation of people with chronic conditions as a means to shift care and resources out of hospitals into the community (Box 2.1).

> **Box 2.1 Cooperating partners within the Østerbro health care centre**
>
> **The citizen** has a pivotal role in the care pathway, based on the assumption that the patient makes her/his own decisions and wishes to improve her/his quality of life.
>
> **The integrated effort for people living with chronic diseases (SIKS) project** has a steering committee, a project management team and four health care professional working groups – one per diagnostic group. The working groups comprise representatives of health professionals from both primary and secondary health care. A special effort has been made to involve general practitioners (GPs); as gatekeepers they play an important role in the rehabilitation process. In addition, a practice consultant has been attached to the health care centre to support collaboration between the hospital, health care centre and GPs. This involves regular disease-focused meetings to support continuing professional development, with training on motivating change and on managing difficult topics with patients.
>
> **The health care centre** comprises health care staff including two physiotherapists, two nurses, a dietician and a secretary. Staff are being provided with education in teaching health promotion and prevention, as well as training on motivating change and managing difficult conversations.
>
> **The local hospital** collaborates closely with the health care centre through regular meetings. These aim to increase competences among health care workers and are generally disease focused.
>
> **GPs** are responsible for the entire rehabilitation process. They examine and treat patients and then refer them to the health care centre.
>
> **Patients associations** collaborate with the health care centre in the areas of diabetes, heart disease and Chronic Obstructive Pulmonary Disease (COPD).
>
> *Source: Sundhedscenter Østerbro 2007.*

The overarching aim of the health care centre is to improve the quality of care delivered to patients with one or more of the four chronic conditions listed earlier and so to reduce the need for hospitalization. The centre ensures the provision of an integrated care pathway to individuals with chronic conditions through an interdisciplinary and intersectoral collaboration. The health care centre further supports patients in the self-management of their condition(s).

Patients are referred to the health care centre by their GP or the hospital. The number of GP referrals to the health care centre has gradually increased: in June 2005, 45% of GPs in Østerbro referred patients to the health care centre, and by late 2006 this figure had increased to 90%. Once at the health care centre, the patient has an introductory meeting with a health care professional, a rehabilitation programme is planned and, at the end, a concluding meeting is held with a health care professional with follow-up interviews (usually by telephone) at one, three, six and twelve months. Every patient has a focal point at the centre. Once treatment is completed a report is send to the GP. Referral criteria and rehabilitation care pathways are based on clinical guidelines, using the best available evidence.

To further support patients, a self-management course called "Learn to live with chronic conditions" is offered to those who have attended a rehabilitation course at the health care centre. It builds on patients' experiences and competences and is an adaptation of the aforementioned Stanford University CDSMP (Lorig 1993), developed collaboratively by the Arthritis Association, the counties of Copenhagen and Ribe (which are different in terms of size, urbanization and organization of the patient education programme), and the National Board of Health.

The cost of rehabilitation programmes at Østerbro health care centre has been estimated at €547 per person for COPD and €700 per person for type 2 diabetes (excluding capital costs). Although the cost–effectiveness of the programmes has not been assessed, it is expected that the rehabilitation programmes will result in fewer hospitalizations over the long term: 80% of patients at the health care centre have no contact with the hospital and only 1% of COPD patients visit the hospital. However, chronic conditions deteriorate over time, and thus rehabilitation programmes may help to prevent progression and thereby prevent subsequent hospitalizations.

A patient journey: Denmark

Patients with chronic conditions are typically diagnosed by a GP. Here we describe a typical patient journey for a fictitious patient: a 54-year-old woman with type 2 diabetes and COPD. She has a leg ulcer and moderate retinopathy. The patient is also moderately obese (body mass index (BMI) of 27). She has been unemployed for three years, receives social assistance benefits, and lives on her own.

In the Danish health care system, patients are not screened for diabetes and therefore the patient may go undiagnosed for a long time. The patient will typically be diagnosed by her GP. According to the new guidelines for COPD, smokers or ex-smokers above 35 years of age who have one or more pulmonary symptoms should be examined by their GPs. This means that the patient will probably be diagnosed with COPD before being diagnosed with diabetes.

After diagnosis of COPD, the severity of the disease will be assessed and follow-up will be carried out regularly by her GP. The aim of this regular follow-up is to support the patient in lifestyle changes and thereby prevent the progression of the disease. Once type 2 diabetes is diagnosed, the GP will evaluate the patient's complications, risk factors and lifestyle, knowledge, attitude and resources. Based on the severity of the disease and the resources of the patient, the GP will decide whether to take on the patient's case or to refer her to a diabetes outpatient clinic, a health care centre (although there are only a few available in Denmark) and/or educational sessions. The GP will also refer the patient to an ophthalmologist and to a privately practising dermatologist if the leg ulcer is severe or does not heal. Several regions in Denmark have shared care agreements between general practice and diabetes outpatient clinics. After the initial treatment phase, there will again be follow-up for the patient in the general practice or at the diabetes outpatient clinic (or both) every third month.

Based on a total assessment of the patient's activity level and the severity of the diseases, the patient will be offered a personalized rehabilitation programme. This might include a smoking cessation course, prescribed exercise at a fitness centre, diet counselling, patient education for COPD and psychosocial support. The family network will be assessed to strengthen the patient's social network and the patient will probably be referred to a social worker. The social worker can help the patient to obtain any necessary equipment and can assess her employment opportunities. Since the patient is unemployed and receives social assistance benefits, her medication costs will be refunded partially by the municipality.

Health system features supporting programmes

Targets, standards and guidelines

A National Indicator Project (NIP), established in 2000, assesses the quality of care provided by hospitals to groups of patients with specific medical conditions (Mainz et al. 2003). It seeks to create awareness among patients, families, doctors, nurses and other health care professionals about the extent to which treatment meets appropriate standards. Data are extracted from medical records on eight frequently occurring conditions (including syncope, diabetes, cardiac failure, lung cancer and schizophrenia) to yield information on severity, treatment and outcomes. The NIP findings are used to identify where improvement is needed and quality data are made available to the public to facilitate comparison and choice (The Danish National Indicator Project 2007). A similar system is being developed for general practice by the Quality Unit for General Practice (Den Almenmedicinske Kvalitetsenhed), comparable to the standards and indicators employed by the Danish National Institute of Quality and Accreditation in Healthcare (Danish Institute for Quality and Accreditation in Healthcare 2008).

Evidence-based guidelines are developed by medical societies and, more recently, nursing associations. For example, the Danish Endocrine Society and the Danish College of General Practitioners both provide clinical guidelines on the treatment of diabetes. The Network of Health Promoting Hospitals in Denmark provides guidelines on the non-pharmacological treatment of chronic conditions, for example, rehabilitation programmes for COPD and cardiovascular diseases. The National Board of Health is developing reference programmes, which define the package of care, covering the entire progression from diagnosis to rehabilitation, as well as including prevention and organizational and financial aspects, for a range of disease processes.

However, despite these activities, little is known about the uptake and use of clinical guidelines in the Danish health care system, although an evaluation of the services provided by GPs to people with chronic conditions in general practice and diabetes clinics is under way. This study will also investigate to what extent clinical information systems are being used in each setting.

Health care workforce and capacity

The number of doctors in Denmark is increasing but at a slightly lower rate than in other countries of the EU, reflecting a failure to expand medical training programmes in the 1970s and 1980s. Thus, recruitment of doctors is increasingly difficult, particularly in rural areas (Strandberg-Larsen et al. 2007). A shortage of nurses is currently the most serious staffing problem facing the Danish health sector, in this case reflecting low salaries and heavy workload. However, the situation is changing and the number of nursing students increased between 2001 and 2005 (Strandberg-Larsen et al. 2007).

There is no requirement for continuous education and training of GPs in the Danish health care system. There has, however, been an expansion of Master's-level courses in areas relevant to chronic disease, such as a Master of Health Pedagogy and a Master of Rehabilitation. A training programme for nurses working in diabetes care has also been established (The Danish Nurses Organisation 2000), and a similar programme is being planned for nurses working with patients who have COPD (Box 2.2).

Financial management and incentives

One of the consequences of the recent structural reform has been a change in the way the health care system is financed. With the replacement of the previous counties, which had raised their own revenue, by regions, health care began to be financed by means of a combination of a national earmarked "health tax", allocated through block grants to regions, and municipality funding. National taxes account for approximately 80% of expenditure at the regional level, with another 20% contributed by municipalities, paid as a combination of per capita contribution and activity-based remuneration. The municipal co-financing is intended to create incentives for municipalities to increase preventative services in order to reduce hospitalization rates. The national health tax aims to create

> **Box 2.2 Goals for the supplementary training of nurses in diabetes care**
>
> - Strengthen and further develop the participants' knowledge and skills in relation to diabetes care in primary, secondary and tertiary health care.
> - Expand the entire health care service for people with diabetes in order to improve the quality of the treatment and to optimize the utilization of resources in the health care system.
> - Develop further the educational skills of nurses to enhance diabetes patients' self-management skills and thereby prevent acute complications and the development of the co-morbidities.
> - Improve the level of nursing quality and ensure ongoing quality assurance of evidence-based practice.
> - Strengthen and expand interdisciplinary and intersectoral collaboration and ensure continuity and homogeneity in diabetes care.
> - Strengthen and expand health promotion and prevention efforts in relation to lifestyle changes and behavioural changes for people at risk of developing diabetes.
>
> *Source: The Danish Nurses Organisation 2000.*

greater transparency for taxpayers regarding health expenditure. The impact of this reform is not yet clear but it has been greeted by a mixture of both optimism and scepticism (Nielsen & Østergaard 2006).

In 2006 a financial incentive was piloted among GPs to improve quality of care for patients with diabetes. The financial incentive takes the form of a fee to be paid, on an annual basis, for covering the various elements of a disease management programme, thus tailoring the care provided to the needs of the patient. This requires the GP to assess regularly the appropriateness of the programme for the individual patient and to document consultations over the course of a year. Follow-up visits must be agreed between the GP and the patient and there is an obligation on the part of the GP to follow up any non-attendance, implying an outreach function that is new for Danish GPs. It also promotes intersectoral collaboration, linking the various services offered in the municipalities, as well as self-management (Danish Regions 2007).

Evaluation and lessons learned

Given that approaches to chronic disease management in Denmark are still largely at an experimental stage, there is as yet little information on their impact. However, several pilots have been, or will soon be, evaluated. For example, the 18 health care centres that are co-funded by the Ministry of the Interior and Health will undergo both a self-evaluation and an external evaluation. The external evaluation is being conducted by the National Institute of Public Health. The aim of the evaluation is to assess the degree of implementation of the concept of the health care centre and, if feasible, to assess the impact of the rehabilitation programmes provided. It also aims to clarify the appropriateness of different health care centre models (Box 2.3).

The Stanford University CDSMP, for example, used at the Østerbro health care centre, has undergone a detailed evaluation. As noted earlier, the CDSMP formed the basis for a self-management support programme. Evaluation was undertaken by an external consultancy agency and focused on whether the programme – originally developed in an American context – would be transferable to the Danish cultural, social and health-related context, looking at relevance, quality of education material and cultural transferability, as well as at organizational aspects.

The evaluation used a mix of quantitative and qualitative methods, involving a survey among programme participants, telephone interviews with instructors being trained, focus groups with (leading) master instructors and one-to-one interviews with cooperation partners from the Arthritis Association, the counties of Copenhagen and Ribe and the National Board of Health. It found high levels of satisfaction among programme participants. The fact that the course instructor was someone with a chronic disease had created the opportunity for an equal dialogue and motivated participants to learn new skills and techniques to manage everyday life with a chronic condition. Based on these findings, and the high level of interest in the patient education concept among patients and health professionals alike, the National Board of Health has recommended that the concept is rolled out on a national basis. Indeed, the National Board of Health has concluded a licence agreement with Stanford University to use the programme and is in the process of establishing an organization to manage the process, including translation and publication

---

Box 2.3 Evaluating the rehabilitation programme at Østerbro health care centre

The evaluation of the Østerbro health care centre is part of a larger evaluation of The integrated effort for people living with chronic diseases (SIKS) project. The evaluation is ongoing, but preliminary findings suggest that the physiotherapy training programmes have had a considerable impact, as assessed by two general measures of functionality. Also, a disease-specific assessment for patients with Chronic Obstructive Pulmonary Disease (COPD) pointed to substantial improvement during the training programme. There was also some evidence pointing to a positive effect of the rehabilitation programme for individuals with type 2 diabetes, as indicated by a reduction in weight and waist measurements, as well as improvements in functionality measures and HbA1c levels.

of education materials, coordination of training of programme instructors and quality assurance mechanisms (National Board of Health 2006).

In general, despite ongoing work introducing performance management approaches and programme evaluations, there are numerous potential barriers to optimizing levels of care for patients with chronic diseases within the Danish health care system. These include staff shortages; heavy workloads; a low priority placed on chronic care by health care professionals; lack of political will; limited data (and experience of data recording); limited resources (including information technology (IT)); professional and political reluctance to undertake screening programmes; and professional resistance to working in interdisciplinary teams (see Table 2.1).

Investing in the future

The 2005 report by the National Board of Health, *Chronic conditions – patient, health care system and society – Prerequisites for the good care pathway*, sets out conditions and actions for improved care for patients with chronic conditions (National Board of Health 2006). The report draws, to some extent, on the CCM mentioned earlier and identifies the following areas for improvement: potential for greater self-management; improved organization of care; the use of decision support systems, such as guidelines and DMPs; a supportive community and policy framework; and implementation of IT systems. The National Board of Health has committed to follow through on a number of recommendations, listed later, and to pursue research and development in this area.

The report recommends that each individual with a chronic condition is supported by the health care system to maximize their potential, with access to education and rehabilitation. These should draw on patients' own experiences, supported by the national roll-out of the Stanford patient education model and the creation of regional networks to facilitate programme delivery and quality assurance.

Overall it places great emphasis on supporting patient self-management, through the provision of appropriate information; the use of telemedicine solutions, such as reminders and instructions; as well as greater use of self-monitoring of disease, supported by new technologies and guidelines and backed up by appropriate financing systems.

The National Board of Health proposes that the organization of the health care system should be adapted better to the special needs of chronic disease management. This includes a focus on the patient, with care being provided mainly in the primary care setting but with good coordination with other sectors and across regions.

Table 2.1. *Chronic disease management in Denmark: strengths and weaknesses*

Strengths	Weaknesses	Opportunities	Threats
Equitable and accessible tax-based health care system	Budgetary constraints	Increased political interest	Competing political priorities in other areas
Access to health care services free at the point of use	Tripartite health care system (municipalities, general practice and hospitals) and resultant conflicting policy goals between the three levels	Local initiatives may result in useful programmes	Lack of resources
			Lack of data
Gatekeeper function for GPs		New collaboration agreements between the sectors	Weak financial incentives
	Lack of demand for ongoing training of GPs		Lack of a national plan for local development
Increasing political interest in chronic disease management	Lack of demand for evaluation GP competences	Implementation of the NIP	Extensive decentralized decision-making
New health care agreements	40% of Danish general practices are single-handed practices, potentially impeding the implementation of guidelines and of technological advances	National IT strategy	Free choice for patients can result in uncoordinated care
Social and health care services are integrated at municipality level		Development of national chronic disease plans and programmes	
	Municipalities have limited competences and resources in the health care arena	New structural reform partially motivated by the needs of chronic disease patients	Health care costs can be excessively high
A high degree of IT in general practice			Relatively high levels of political attention focused on elective surgery and cancer
A high degree of patient choice (GP and hospital)	Staff shortages	Citizens have greater opportunities to access health-related information and knowledge	
	Care for people with chronic conditions not considered prestigious among health care professionals		Demographic changes may imply that treating chronic diseases will become excessively expensive, so that offering good health care services to the entire population will be challenging
	Political focus on waiting lists diverts attention from chronic conditions towards elective surgery		
	Limited data on clinical practice and chronic disease burden		
	GPs' reluctance to be involved in interdisciplinary teams		

Source: Authors' own compilation.

Notes: GP: General practitioner; IT: Information technology; NIP: National Indicator Project.

It further supports interdisciplinary working, drawing on the professional skills of nurses and other health care workers, in collaboration with GPs and patients. It does, however, see the GP as the person who navigates the patient through the entire care pathway. It also envisages a new type of worker, the "case manager" who can assist those patients with poor understanding of their disease or those that are unable to adhere to treatment and recommended lifestyle changes. The case manager can be based in general practice, in the municipal health care system or in a hospital department. The National Board of Health also made a series of recommendations aiming to strengthen information collection methods.

In recognition of the value of intersectoral working, the National Board of Health argues that the local community should motivate patients to pursue active self-management and should facilitate healthy lifestyles. Health professionals should thus work with staff from the social sector, patients associations, training organizations, leisure organizations and other relevant public and private organizations.

In summary, it is only recently that a strategy for chronic conditions has been developed within the Danish health care system. The work has been driven largely by the National Board of Health and several committed individuals from the health care system throughout the country, with the Ministry of Interior and Health providing funding for its development. Since it is usually clinicians and researchers that drive developments in Danish health care, it is unusual that chronic care initiatives are now being led by the country's central administration. It will thus be interesting to see how this new model evolves.

References

Bodenheimer T, Wagner EH, Grumbach K (2002). Improving primary care for patients with chronic illness. *Journal of the American Medical Association*, 288:1775–1779.

Danish Institute for Quality and Accreditation in Healthcare (2008) [web site]. Institut for Kvalitet og Akkreditering i Sundhedsvæsenet [Danish Institute for Quality and Accreditation in Healthcare]. Århus, Danish Institute for Quality and Accreditation in Healthcare (http://www.kvalitetsinstitut.dk/, accessed May 2008).

Danish Regions (2007) [web site]. Copenhagen, Danish Regions (www.regioner.dk, accessed November 2007).

Jensen CR, Borg E, Kofoed BG (2007). *Østerbro Sundhedscenter – fra idé til drift* [Østerbro Health Care Centre – from idea to operation]. Copenhagen, The Health Care Administration, Municipality of Copenhagen.

Lorig K (1993). Self-management of chronic illness: a model for the future. *Generations*, 17:11–14.

Mainz J et al. (2003). Nationwide continuous quality improvement using clinical indicators: the Danish National Indicator Project. *International Journal for Quality in Health Care*, 16:45–50.

Ministry of the Interior and Health (2003). *Healthy throughout life – the targets and strategies for public health policy of the Government of Denmark, 2002–2010.* Copenhagen, Ministry of the Interior and Health.

National Board of Health (2004). *National Board of Health Project on major noncommunicable diseases*. Copenhagen, Danish National Board of Health.

National Board of Health (2006). *Chronic conditions – Patients, health care and community*. Copenhagen, National Board of Health.

Nielsen AJ et al. (2006). *Sundhedspersonalets rådgivning om sundhedsadfærd – En kortlægning og analyse [Health personnel advice on health behaviour – mapping and analysis]*. Copenhagen, Danish Institute for Health Services Research.

Nielsen ML, Østergaard M (2006). *Udlægning af genoptræning – Fra sygehus til kommuner [Interpretation of rehabilitation – from the hospital to the municipality]*. Copenhagen, Danish Institute for Health Services Research.

Strandberg-Larsen M et al. (2007). Denmark: Health system review. *Health Systems in Transition*, 9(6);1–162.

The Danish National Indicator Project (2007) [web site]. The Danish National Indicator Project. Århus, The Danish National Indicator Project (http://www.nip.dk, accessed 13 August 2008).

The Danish Nurses Organisation (2000). *Længerevarende efteruddannelse for sygeplejersker i diabetessygepleje [Long-term continuing education of nurses in diabetes care]*. Copenhagen, The Danish Nurses Organisation.

Willaing I, Folmann N, Gisselbaek A (2005). *Patientskoler og gruppebaseret undervisning - en litteraturgennemgang med fokus på metoder og effekter [Patient schools and group based education - a literature review focusing on methods and effects]*. Copenhagen, National Board of Health.

Chapter 3
England

Debra de Silva, Daragh Fahey

Context

In England[1], health services are provided predominantly through a tax-funded National Health Service (NHS), which is 60 years old in 2008. All NHS-funded health care, except dentistry, optometry and prescriptions, is free at the point of use. The planning and delivery system is hierarchical, with the Department of Health and government offices providing a policy focus and 10 Strategic Health Authorities (SHAs) providing strategic leadership at regional level. Approximately 80% of the entire budget is devolved to 152 geographically defined primary care trusts (PCTs), which in many parts of the country are co-terminous with local government districts (including social services), but are independent of them. The PCTs are responsible for purchasing services from all health providers, within a detailed framework, encompassing standards and targets set out by the Department of Health and monitored on its behalf by the SHAs.

The ruling political party sets health care policy. The Department (Ministry) of Health, which is responsible for the funding and operation of the NHS, is headed by a cabinet minister. Improving health care is high on the current political agenda, and there has been significant investment in improving access to services in recent years. As in other countries, the increasing age of the population and the growing burden of chronic disease have created pressure on costs. In response, the Government has prioritized more spending on disease

---
1. In the United Kingdom, the responsibility for health care is devolved to England, Scotland, Northern Ireland and Wales. Consequently, the organization of health care differs in the devolved countries.

prevention, health promotion and schemes to increase self-care and community care. The aim is to shift service provision from secondary care to primary care where feasible, based on the assumption that health services can be provided more cost-effectively in primary care (Department of Health 2006a).

Primary health care teams, including GPs, nurses and other health workers, provide most primary health care services; usually in community-based health centres. Everyone legally resident in the United Kingdom is eligible to register for free with a GP. General practice services are commissioned by PCTs based on a nationally negotiated contract. GPs have also been given increased power to commission services, as part of government policy to provide enhanced community and patient-oriented services ("practice-based commissioning") (Department of Health 2004a). Salaried staff within hospitals provide secondary and tertiary care. Organizations delivering health care, whether in hospitals or the community (as with mental health), are termed "trusts". Hospital trusts negotiate reimbursement with the local PCT and GP commissioning groups based on nationally agreed activity-based tariffs ("Payment by Results").

In addition to publicly provided NHS health care, there is a growing number of private providers. These traditionally offered supplementary care and were paid for from personal or employer-provided insurance or direct payment by the patient. However, the Government's policy of increasing competition has led to a growing volume of NHS-funded care being delivered by independent (private) providers.

Social care services (social welfare) are distinct from health in most areas. Although some integrated health and social care trusts exist, it is usual for social services to be provided by local government.

Analysing the response

Approaches to chronic disease management

A variety of service models have been implemented for people with chronic conditions in England (these are often referred to as long-term conditions in official documents). This section provides an overview of some of the key components of the generic NHS model.

In January 2005 the Government launched a bespoke NHS Health and Social Care Model designed to help health and social care organizations improve care for people with long-term conditions (Department of Health 2005a) (Fig. 3.1). This model builds on approaches such as the Chronic Care Model (CCM) originating in the United States and a number of policy initiatives in

Fig. 3.1 *The National Health Service and Social Care Long-Term Conditions Model*

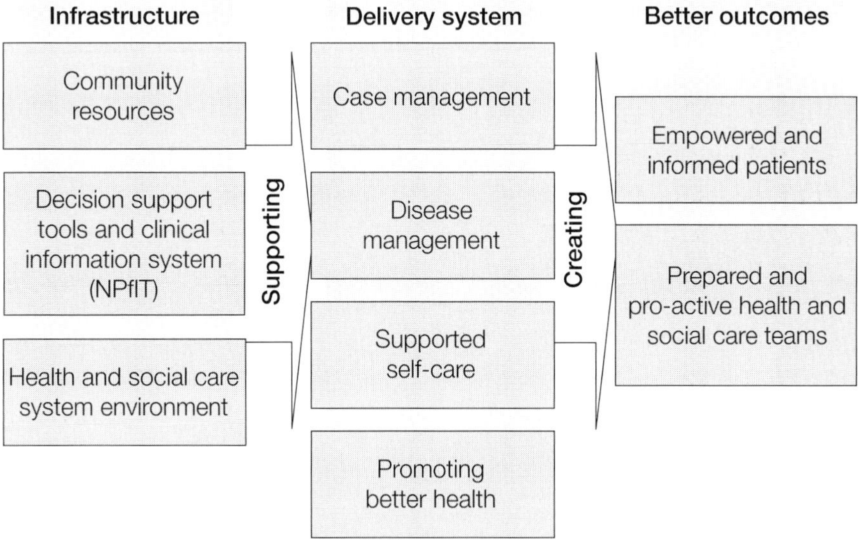

Infrastructure	Delivery system	Better outcomes
Community resources	Case management	Empowered and informed patients
Decision support tools and clinical information system (NPfIT)	Disease management	Prepared and pro-active health and social care teams
Health and social care system environment	Supported self-care	
	Promoting better health	

(Supporting / Creating)

Source: Department of Health 2005a.

England such as the NHS Improvement Plan (Department of Health 2004b) and the NHS Chronic Disease Management "Compendium of Information" (Department of Health 2004c). A full history of the development of policy in this area is beyond the scope of this chapter, but England has recognized the need to develop chronic care services since the late 1990s.

The NHS and Social Care Model focuses on how people with long-term conditions will be identified so they can receive care according to their needs. It describes how an "Expert Patients Programme" will be expanded to promote peer-led education in self-management; how specialist nurses (termed "community matrons") will support people with complex conditions (see later); and how teams of staff will be encouraged to work together with people with long-term conditions and their families. The key facets of the model are:

- a systematic approach that links health, social care, service users and carers;
- identifying everyone with a long-term condition;
- stratifying people so they can receive care according to their needs;
- focusing on frequent users of secondary care services;

- using community matrons to carry out case management;
- developing ways to identify people who may become very high-intensity service users;
- establishing multidisciplinary teams in primary care, supported by specialist advice;
- developing local methods to support self-care;
- expanding self-management education programmes such as the Expert Patient Programme;
- using tools and techniques already available to make an impact.

The stated principles driving this approach include improvement in the quality and accessibility of care for people with long-term conditions and containment or reduction of the costs associated with chronic care.

In January 2006 a White Paper entitled *Our health, our care, our say: a new direction for community services* set out the Government's vision for community-based care (Department of Health 2006a). While not focused exclusively on people with long-term conditions, this is a key driver of how chronic care is being redesigned. The aim is to shift care from being delivered reactively, often in a hospital setting, towards more responsive community-based services. This involves far more than changing the location where care is delivered. Instead, it involves a whole system change, including behavioural and attitudinal changes among service users and professionals (Department of Health 2007).

What differentiated the White Paper from earlier policy documents was that it was based on an extensive consultative process. Public events and meetings with stakeholders were used to shape the key components of future plans. In particular, people said that they wanted health and social care to work together or be more "joined up", that they wanted to receive more care closer to home, and that they wanted services that would help them maintain their independence. Related documents, such as a new commissioning framework for health and social care, build on this approach (Department of Health 2007a).

A number of reviews have been undertaken to support the NHS in understanding different models of care and to help define the critical success factors related to new approaches (Hutt, Rosen & McCauley 2004, Singh 2005a, Singh 2005b). The Department of Health continues to examine the types of activity and workforce capacity needed to improve chronic disease management, but we identified little publicly available evidence of modelling being utilized to examine the suitability of the approaches already in place in England, or possible alternatives.

Distribution, uptake and coverage

While the Government has provided an overarching vision for chronic care services, implementation has varied, with service delivery models being applied at local, regional and national levels. A 2006 survey of England's SHAs, which are responsible for overseeing service provision on a regional basis, found that most did not report any particular model guiding the implementation of services for people with long-term conditions (Singh & Ham 2006). One third reported that a regional model had been adopted, such as the CCM or adaptations of the population management ("pyramid of care") approach developed by the United States health provider Kaiser Permanente. Elsewhere, the agenda was being driven by individual PCTs. As a consequence, approaches to chronic disease management vary widely in each part of the country. However, there are some common core elements, including a focus on self-management education; nurse-led clinics and other nurse-led services; multidisciplinary teams, including joint working between health and social services; shifting services from hospital settings into the community; risk stratification, sometimes using computer modelling of primary and secondary care data; and case management, including specialist nurses (community matrons). Many other service delivery models are being implemented in individual localities.

Just as the range of approaches varies in different parts of England, so too does the scope of these approaches. Government policies are both generalist, focusing on people with long-term conditions as a group, and specific, with approaches targeted at improving care for people with specific conditions and people who use services frequently. Although some initiatives focus on people aged 65 and over (see Box 3.1), the general approach is to acknowledge that people from many age groups are affected by long-term conditions and age is just one among many factors for targeting services. We identified no countrywide (within England) frameworks for working with children with long-term conditions or people from minority ethnic groups, although individualized services for these groups have been developed in some places.

One challenge for local and regional approaches has been the 2006 reorganization of PCTs and SHAs throughout England. Organizations were merged and their roles altered somewhat. The number of PCTs and SHAs was reduced from, respectively, 302 to 152 and from 28 to 10, thus increasing the size of health regions. As a consequence, local and regional delivery models had to be readjusted to accommodate this new structure, in some cases leading to existing programmes being disbanded.

> **Box 3.1 East Sussex "Independence First" Partnerships for Older People Projects**
>
> The East Sussex "Independence First" project was set up in 2006 within the Government's Partnership for Older People Project (POPP), which aims to foster joint working between health and social services. Independence First is a partnership between East Sussex County Council, local health and social services teams, and community and voluntary services. The goal was to integrate both preventative and specialized care into a coherent service package to help older people remain at home and independent.
>
> Within this service model, case finding tools and referral from health professionals are used to identify older people who may benefit from extra support. Those judged to be at high risk of hospitalization are directed to community matron services, while those at lower risk are assessed by a navigation service operated by the voluntary sector. Both navigators and community matrons may refer service users to specialist services as required. These include a memory assessment team, intensive home support teams, falls specialists, medicines management support, a single point of access for the acute care/community hospital interface, osteoporosis services, delivery and fitting of simple aids and equipment, and social care.
>
> Innovative aspects of this model include integration (health and social services working together, council administering finances); substituting skills (using the voluntary sector as navigators); substituting the location of care (home- and community-based services); segmenting service users into high- and lower-risk groups; and new types of service delivery (navigators, and pharmacists visiting people at home).
>
> Following a 2-year pilot, successful components of Independence First are being integrated into the routine practice of social and health care agencies. Impacts on clinical indicators, staff perceptions, service use (including admission rates), and participants' health status and quality of life are being assessed – and have shown favourable outcomes to date. The most significant challenge has been identifying appropriate case finding tools to allow referral for preventive services.

Community matrons in England

The NHS Improvement Plan describes a new role for nurses working in chronic disease management (Department of Health 2004b). Community matrons are senior nurses who use case management techniques to support high-intensity users of health care or people at high risk of hospitalization. In 2005 the Department of Health instructed all SHAs to implement a community matron strategy, providing guidance regarding the number required in each area, based on demographic and health services information and agreed implementation measures to be incorporated in local delivery plans.

Community matrons are central to the Government's policy for supporting people with long-term conditions, with 3000 community matrons due to have been in post by March 2007 (Department of Health 2005b). They are seen as a key provider and procurer of care, responsible for ensuring that all health and social care needs are met. They also seek to support self-management, with the overall aim being to support people so they can remain at home longer and avoid or delay admission to hospital or other institutions. PCTs have assumed ongoing responsibility for funding the initiative and they also have to report to the Department of Health on the number of community matrons in post.

Although community matrons work in different ways throughout England, there are some commonalities. They tend to be nurses or therapists based in primary care settings, tasked with coordinating primary and secondary care and social services. In large part, community matrons have been recruited from the existing pool of primary care nurses. Most will undergo advanced clinical and case management training, offered by universities or private providers. National competency frameworks and guidance on training have been developed (NHS Modernisation Agency and Skills for Health 2005, Department of Health 2006c).

Community matrons aim to use standardized risk assessment tools to identify people who may benefit from support and undertake detailed assessments. Increasingly, they are working alongside pharmacists to review medication. The key components of this model are:

- segmentation of people at high risk of admission or frequent service users;
- use of clinical information systems to identify people at high risk;
- simplification of care pathways (by having one person coordinating other services);
- supporting self-management and individualized care planning;
- ongoing case management, often for an extended period.

There has been little evaluation of the community matron strategy as yet, although a national pilot found that advanced nurses may not significantly reduce unplanned admissions (Boaden et al. 2005, Gravelle et al. 2007). PCTs have also been assessing the impacts of community matrons on hospital admissions. Early evidence is mixed: in some areas community matrons have had little impact on overall admission rates, whereas others report admissions being avoided (South Yorkshire Academy for Health and Care Improvement 2006). Areas where community matrons have been most successful appear to be those where the role is implemented as a part of a broader chronic disease management programme, integrated with other services.

One of the main concerns about how chronic care strategies will affect the workforce is the impact of community matrons on district nursing. There is evidence that many community matrons are being recruited from the already limited pool of district nurses (NHS National Workforce Projects, 2006). However, there is also evidence that community matrons are largely fulfilling the work of district nurses, but not doing much extra.

A patient journey: England

To illustrate current practice within the NHS, we describe a "typical patient journey" for Jane, a 54-year-old woman with type 2 diabetes and COPD, who has a leg ulcer and moderate retinopathy. Jane is also moderately obese, unemployed and lives alone.

While services and protocols may vary in different parts of the country, Jane's COPD would typically be diagnosed by her GP when she presents with symptoms of COPD (increasing breathlessness and coughing) or a respiratory infection and a history of moderate to heavy smoking. Alternatively, she may present to the local hospital Accident and Emergency Department. The GP or hospital clinician would diagnose COPD based on history, examination and some basic investigations such as a chest X-ray and pulmonary function tests.

If Jane first presented to primary care for diagnosis of COPD, her GP is more likely to try to manage her disease rather than refer her to secondary care. Jane would probably be referred to a practice nurse for smoking cessation services, given a prescription for an inhaler or nicotine patches and/or referred for pulmonary rehabilitation. In cases of uncertainty or difficulty managing symptoms, Jane's GP would refer her to hospital for specialist care. If Jane initially presented to the hospital Accident and Emergency Department she would commonly be referred to the hospital respiratory physicians for initial management.

Type 2 diabetes is typically asymptomatic in its early stages. Jane's diabetes would probably have been picked up opportunistically as part of a routine glucose screening test offered to those who are overweight. GPs and practice nurses are increasingly likely to manage diabetes themselves but some will seek an initial assessment in secondary care. The clinician will confirm the diagnosis and look for evidence of complications of the disease in addition to giving advice on management. Jane would likely be referred to a dietician (to lose weight and optimize diet), a chiropodist (for ulcers), and an ophthalmologist or some other diabetic retinopathy screening or monitoring service. She may need to attend a pharmacist for medication to control the level of glucose and a phlebotomist for blood tests. Initiation of insulin might take place during a hospital outpatient appointment, undertaken by a specialist nurse.

Jane's care for her diabetes and her COPD would largely be seen as separate care pathways (Fig. 3.2), although initiatives in some local areas support a more integrated approach.

England   **37**

Fig. 3.2 *A patient journey in England*

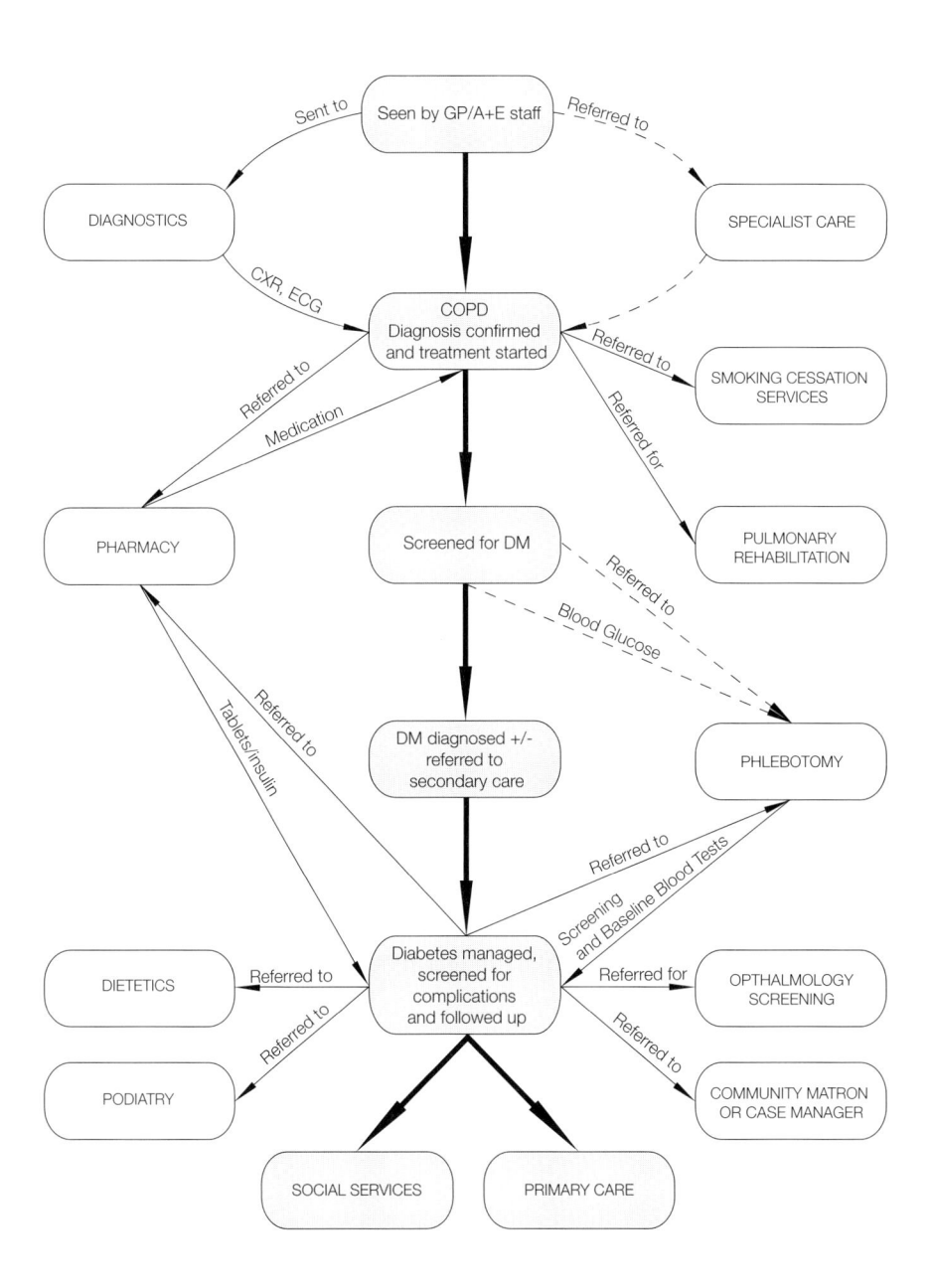

Source: Authors' own compilation.

Notes: A&E: Accident and Emergency Department; DM: Diabetes mellitus; CXR: Chest X-ray; ECG: Electrocardiogram.

Jane is unemployed so she will already have been in contact with social services about welfare benefits. If Jane's condition worsens as she gets older she may experience failing sight and increasing breathlessness. In this case, Jane, her family, or health care professionals would probably notify social services (local government), which would trigger the release of a number of care options, such as district nursing (to care for her ulcer), general carers (to provide basic home care), occupational therapist assessment, "meals on wheels" (meals prepared and delivered daily to her home), increased social security financial benefits (particularly if registered blind) and access to a number of day care support centres. As Jane's condition deteriorates, a case manager would probably be assigned to coordinate Jane's care, either from the social or health services. In some regions she would have access to special end-of-life health care services.

Health system features supporting programmes

Targets, standards and guidelines

The Government in England has established some countrywide targets for improving care for people with long-term conditions. For example, all health care organizations are required to reduce the number of days spent in hospital following emergency admissions by 5% by 2008; targets have been set for the roll-out of self-management education programmes; PCTs have been set a recruitment target for community matrons to provide complex case management; National Service Frameworks (NSFs) have set standards and service targets for a variety of conditions; the QOF rewards GPs for achieving a package of care elements; and a pharmacy contract rewards annual reviews of use of medicines as well as other proactive checks.

These initiatives are monitored centrally, with health organizations required to report regularly on progress. However, we identified no centralized records regarding the overall number and distribution of chronic care initiatives in England, nor the percentage of providers taking part in different types of initiatives.

NSFs provide evidence-based guidance on certain chronic diseases (Box 3.2). They set measurable goals and national standards, and identify key interventions for a defined service or care group. They also set out strategies to support implementation and ensure progress within an agreed time frame.

Each NSF is developed with the assistance of an external reference group which includes health professionals, service users, carers, health service managers, partner agencies and others, supported by the Department of Health. At the time of writing NSFs address diabetes, heart disease, cancer, renal disease, mental health, children, older people, paediatric intensive care and long-term

> **Box 3.2 Standards for the National Service Framework for diabetes**
>
> Standard 1 (Prevention of type 2 diabetes) on strategies to reduce type 2 diabetes risk in the general population and reduce inequalities in type 2 diabetes risk.
>
> Standard 2 (Identification of people with diabetes) on strategies to identify people who do not know they have diabetes.
>
> Standard 3 (Empowering people with diabetes) on encouraging partnership in decision-making, diabetes management and adoption of a healthy lifestyle.
>
> Standard 4 (Clinical care of adults with diabetes) on ensuring high-quality care for adults.
>
> Standards 5 & 6 (Clinical care of children and young people with diabetes) on ensuring high-quality care for children and young people.
>
> Standard 7 (Management of diabetic emergencies) on protocols for rapid and effective treatment of diabetic emergencies by appropriately trained health care professionals.
>
> Standard 8 (Care of people with diabetes during admission to hospital) on ensuring effective diabetes care in hospital and continued patient involvement in diabetes management.
>
> Standard 9 (Diabetes and pregnancy) on policies to optimize pregnancy outcomes in women with pre-existing diabetes and those who develop diabetes during pregnancy.
>
> Standards 10, 11 & 12 (Detection and management of long-term complications) on regular surveillance for the long-term complications of diabetes.
>
> *Source: Adapted from Department of Health 2001.*

neurological conditions, amongst others. NHS organizations are expected to report their performance against these NSFs.

The 2005 Long-term (Neurological) Conditions NSF has the following key themes: independent living; care planned around the needs and choices of the individual; easier, timely access to services; and joint working across all agencies and disciplines involved. This NSF encourages intersectoral action to support people living independently by providers of transport, housing, employment, education, benefits and pensions, among others.

The NSFs build on evidence-based guidelines prepared by the National Institute for Health and Clinical Excellence (NICE) and other public and private bodies, such as the Royal Colleges (representing physicians), including the National Collaborating Centre for Chronic Conditions (National Collaborating Centre for Chronic Conditions 2007), professional organizations and others. The Department of Health commissions NICE to provide evidence-based guidelines to inform research-based practice (NICE 2007). NICE also provides tools to help managers and health professionals implement guidance, such as commissioning guides, cost templates, and audit criteria.

In addition to documents supporting Department of Health policy, many national organizations have produced material to support chronic disease management. These include NHS organizations such as the NHS Integrated Service Improvement Programme (ISIP) (ISIP 2007), the NHS Institute for Innovation and Improvement (NHS Institute for Innovation and Improvement 2007) and NHS Networks (NHS Networks 2007), as well as independent think tanks and academic institutes and universities.

Decision support systems tend to be developed locally, although the nationally developed Patients At Risk of Re-hospitalization (PARR) tool is available to help with risk stratification (Billings et al. 2006).

Health care workforce and capacity

The NHS is increasingly commissioning the private sector for certain services such as telecare and orthopaedic clinics. As from 2005, the private sector is expected to provide additional NHS-subsidized diagnostic procedures at an estimated worth of £1 billion over five years, with an estimated 1.5 million NHS-subsidized diagnostic tests per annum (Department of Health 2006d). However, most professionals caring for individuals with long-term conditions are based in the public sector, including practice and specialist nurses working in primary care, family doctors, GPs with special interests (GPwSI), hospital doctors and nurses, mental health practitioners, pharmacists, emergency care practitioners, paramedics and other allied heath professionals.

Some roles, such as that of community matron, have been developed specifically to address the needs of people with long-term conditions. Other roles, such as GPwSI are focusing on people with certain long-term conditions, although these roles are not exclusive to the chronic care agenda. The NHS is increasingly working jointly with professionals in social services, the voluntary sector and people with long-term conditions themselves in delivering services. For example, a joint social care and health performance framework is being developed, and pharmacies are becoming a venue for health promotion and smoking cessation services.

The Department of Health has, in recent years, identified workforce development as a critical element of chronic care. In 2002 the NHS "Skills for Health" organization was established to help create a skilled and flexible health care workforce by developing national workforce competency frameworks (for example, for case managers and community matrons), as well as mechanisms for increasing skill levels and promoting qualifications and career frameworks (Skills for Health 2008). It contributes to the expansion of the role(s) of other staff, such as pharmacists, in the chronic disease management agenda. These developments are supported by guidance on education and training commissioned by PCTs and other agencies (Department of Health 2006c).

The NHS has also produced a long-term conditions workforce resource pack to support workforce planning (NHS National Workforce Projects 2006). It provides an overview of current developments, along with a range of practical solutions and examples of good practice. Moreover, NHS organizations have been invited to take part in initiatives to support large-scale workforce change. For example, NHS Employers, which acts for trusts in England on workforce issues, ran a programme with 26 organizational teams from 66 organizations across health care, social care, and the voluntary sector to develop and implement new roles and ways of working to improve services for people with long-term conditions (NHS Employers 2006a). Significant benefits for people with long-term conditions, host organizations and NHS staff were reported.

England has attempted to ensure that health care staff are appropriately remunerated using the "Agenda for Change" policy initiative, whereby the job roles of all non-doctors within the NHS are reviewed to ensure they are paid for the work carried out rather than according to job titles (NHS Employers 2006b).

The Government has created clinical leadership roles to support chronic disease management, most notably "Tsars" or Clinical Directors who should influence, champion and support the implementation of chronic disease policy nationally. They are also appointed for specific diseases such as diabetes and heart disease and to represent groups such as older people and children.

As previously noted, people with long-term conditions themselves are increasingly viewed as a crucial component of the chronic care "workforce." Strategies to support self-management vary in different parts of England and include, for example, projects to help people purchase the services and resources they want by allocating them an annual budget to use as they choose ("individual budgets") (Care Services Improvement Partnership 2006). These strategies are supported by efforts to provide accessible information materials and initiatives such as the Expert Patients Programme (Department of Health 2005c, EPPCIC 2007). However, peer support and self-management education are not routine elements of care. Although providers are encouraged to involve people with long-term conditions actively in decision-making and care planning, support by service providers for self-management varies, reflecting local initiatives, as there are currently no national policies, templates or systems to support them.

Financial management and incentives

Although there has been a recent focus on chronic disease management in England, minimal additional financial resources have been allocated specifically to implement chronic disease management policies. For example, there is no budget specifically allocated to implement the NHS and Social Care Model.

Financial resources are interwoven into the broader payment system. PCTs receive a capitation payment for every resident. This is not linked to chronic disease prevalence, but is adjusted for age and levels of deprivation. PCTs use their annual budgets to reimburse GPs according to nationally agreed contracts. PCTs reimburse hospitals through contracts based on activity levels at nationally agreed tariffs. Individuals with long-term conditions receive no financial incentives or reimbursements for participating in chronic care initiatives nationally.

In 2004 the Treasury (Ministry of Finance) reviewed all NHS spending and identified chronic disease management as a priority (HM Treasury 2004). However, it did not indicate how much individual PCTs should spend, leaving PCTs with the challenge of identifying resources from within current budgets.

The main financial incentives for chronic disease management are focused on primary care. In 2004 England's "GP contract" changed, with the work of a GP became more strictly defined and costed. GPs are expected to provide essential (core) services involving the care and management of those who are ill or think they are ill, and the general management of the terminally ill. Everything else is deemed "non-core" and split into additional and enhanced services. Additional clinical services include the management of certain long-term conditions. If a GP does not wish to or cannot provide these services, they can "opt out". Such services will then need to be provided by the PCT, perhaps by using another general practice or by a community service. Enhanced services are extra services, such as minor surgery, which general practices may choose to implement. These can be locally decided or based on national terms and conditions (Department of Health 2003). The main sources of income in general practice are:

- core service payments – a global sum paid based on the number of people registered with the practice and adjusted for factors which affect workload (such as age, gender, morbidity and mortality);

- enhanced service payments, negotiated between practices and the PCT – groups of practices may come together to provide a set of enhanced services within a catchment area;

- payments for target activity levels, set out through the national Quality and Outcomes Framework (QOF).

The QOF provides financial rewards for "good performance" based on a range of clinical and organizational indicators (Box 3.3). It is not a measure of independently evaluated quality as such, but rather a marker of the achievement of certain activity targets, such as annual reviews of blood pressure or providing smoking cessation advice. This information is collected in a national database system (The Information Centre for Health and Social Care 2007).

Although in theory this approach had merits, in reality most practices were already achieving a points score close to the maximum when the QOF was first introduced. The result is that much more money than expected was paid to GPs in the first year, with limited evidence of improved outcomes (Downing et al. 2007, Khunti et al. 2007, Smith et al. 2008). As a result, the QOF has been revised to increase the expected performance standards in some areas (British Medical Association and NHS Employers 2006).

Another key driver in chronic disease management is the recent policy of "practice-based commissioning", which expects general practices to purchase health services. The rationale is that this may lead to better services for those with long-term conditions if local people influence their primary care clinicians to provide more appropriate care, closer to home. This is encouraged by policies that encourage more coordination between health and social care and joint commissioning of services (Department of Health 2006a).

The financial incentives acting on primary care seek to encourage a preventive approach, whereby people with long-term conditions are provided care within

---

Box 3.3 Domains of reward in the Quality and Outcomes Framework

Practices are awarded points up to a maximum of 1050 points, according to four domains.

Clinical domain: 76 indicators in 11 areas – coronary heart disease; left ventricular disease; stroke or transient ischaemic attack; hypertension; diabetes; Chronic Obstructive Pulmonary Disease (COPD); epilepsy; hypothyroidism; cancer; mental health; and asthma. This domain accounts for up to 550 points and aims to reward adherence to evidence-based guidelines for long-term conditions.

Organizational domain: 56 indicators in 5 areas – records and information about patients; patient communication, education and training; practice management; and medicine management.

Patient experience domain: 4 indicators in 2 areas: patient surveys and consultation length.

Additional services domain: 10 indicators in 4 areas: cervical screening; child health surveillance; maternity services; and contraceptive services.

Source: The Information Centre for Health and Social Care 2007.

their homes and local community, so as to avoid hospital admissions. However, this conflicts with policies to encourage market-oriented provider payments, particularly with regard to secondary care. One such scheme is "Payment by Results", whereby secondary care providers are reimbursed for their activity according to nationally agreed tariffs. The rationale is that this will ensure a fair and consistent basis for hospital funding, rather than being reliant on historic budgets and the negotiating skills of individual managers. However, as hospitals are paid per admission and per number of "extra" days that individuals stay in hospital, this payment system can be expected to encourage hospitals to admit people, carry out more procedures and keep them in hospital for longer, rather than encouraging a preventive approach. The authors could not identify any detailed evaluations which assessed the impacts of these financial policies.

Evaluation and lessons learned

The chronic disease management initiatives being implemented in England are many, varied, and not always coordinated. There are initiatives operating at national level, such as the community matrons system, the NHS Health and Social Care Model, NSFs, and policies to shift more care into the community. There are also regionally based programmes and a large number of localized initiatives, such as nurse telephone follow-up, direct access to diagnostics for GPs, and initiation of insulin in primary care rather than in outpatient settings. Just as the initiatives are varied, so too are the evaluation strategies.

The authors identified no plans to evaluate the NHS Health and Social Care Model as a whole. However, the Department of Health is reviewing its pilot projects and early implementation sites related to the Model (Department of Health 2006b, Department of Health 2006e).

Some of the larger national and regional initiatives have collected "before and after" data or used comparison groups to assess effectiveness during pilot phases. Most of these evaluations have found little reduction in hospital admissions (Boaden et al. 2005). For example, a national evaluation of the community matrons pilots found that while service users were satisfied with case management, the service did not reduce emergency admissions to hospital (Boaden et al. 2006). The evaluation found no evidence of systematic redesign of care and suggested that there was poor liaison between primary and secondary care, sometimes in addition to poor access to community services, and out-of-hours services were not focused on keeping patients out of hospital. The evaluators concluded that more radical system redesign is needed if case management is to have a greater impact on admissions (Gravelle et al. 2007).

Similarly, a national process evaluation of implementation of the Expert Patients self-management education programme in England identified a number of organizational barriers (National Primary Care Research and Development Centre 2005). PCTs were generally not using the goodwill and experience of participants to increase public involvement in local health debates or initiatives and the PCTs tended to be poor at managing tutors because they had little experience of working with volunteers. The evaluation found that professionals were not engaged in the process, were poorly informed about course content and seldom referred people to courses. Most participants were satisfied with the courses but expressed interest in ongoing support or communication. A randomized trial to assess effectiveness is ongoing at the time of writing (Bower et al. 2006).

Evaluations of national initiatives, such as joint social care and health prevention programmes, individual budgets and projects to accelerate shifting care out of hospitals are under way at the time of writing. Evaluations of local services are also ongoing in order to assess the impact of chronic disease management initiatives on patient experience, processes and resource use (NHS Networks 2007). For example, an orthopaedic triage service in Trent found a 12% reduction in referrals to secondary care over the course of one year. A COPD self-management and community care programme in Yorkshire was associated with a readmission rate of 7.8% compared to the national average of 30% (Parker 2006).

One of the key barriers to evaluation may be a lack of experience and confidence in working with data. Feedback from some pilot programmes suggests that managers and practitioners may be eager to evaluate initiatives but are concerned that IT systems or data analysis protocols are not in place and that they do not have the necessary skills to extract, interpret or apply relevant data (Ham et al. 2006).

Although the Department of Health and PCTs are supposed to monitor and assess individual initiatives, and to link detailed performance measures to reimbursement, as yet there is no national strategy to evaluate chronic disease models as a whole or in terms of their impact on the health and social care system.

Reviews of NHS experience and published evidence identify certain critical success factors (Table 3.1).

A learning point is the challenge caused by potentially competing policy frameworks. For example, although the focus of the NHS Health and Social Care Model is on prevention, supporting self-management, and partnership working, in some areas the "Payment by Results" policy may inhibit a change to more community-based care, as it is not in the hospital's financial interest to have more people cared for within the community. This is particularly true for some of the larger hospitals that have been awarded "Foundation Trust" status, giving them greater financial and management autonomy and which are set up to make a profit. "Payment by Results" does allow communities to develop their own local tariffs, and some communities have used this opportunity to develop local tariffs to create incentives for more community-based care for people with long-term conditions.

Another area of concern is the potential for inequitable access to services for people with long-term conditions, as access depends on where people live. This is partly because commissioners have considerable flexibility over which services they decide to offer to their population, and partly because some regions have more resources and capacity to deliver high-quality services. Access to preventive services is particularly variable. Some parts of England are trialling proactive telephone care management for people with long-term conditions, whereas in other areas this service is not available. Most regions are targeting people perceived to be at high risk of hospitalization as a first priority. This approach is driven by the cost of each hospitalization, which is based on a high nationally agreed tariff.

Access for people from ethnic minorities is also being considered in some areas but no countrywide strategic guidance for maintaining equity of access was identified. This is a potential concern given that those from south Asian and black communities are more likely to experience certain long-term conditions but may be less likely to seek treatment or to receive optimal care. As England focuses increasingly on supporting self-care, questions must be asked about whether these services are equally accessible and attractive to people from a wide range of ethnic and sociodemographic groups.

Table 3.1 Critical success factors for chronic disease programmes in England

Whole systems approaches	Training to support staff in new roles, including project management training
Shared boundaries and vision between health and social care	
Empowering people to take responsibility, including service users	Increasing staff competencies
	Organizational stability
Providing care based on levels of need (risk stratification)	High-quality information management and technology
Not running (competing) services in parallel	Involvement of all key stakeholders, including professional representative bodies
Changing professional attitudes and behaviours via organizational culture change	Creating the right incentives
	Adequate investment in services
Overcoming resistance to clinical and managerial change	Adequate time frames in which to test services
Strong clinical leadership	Focusing on realistic targets
	Not assuming that initiatives will reduce costs

Sources: Parker 2006, Singh 2006.

Investing in the future

The lessons learned from current policies and their implementation in England have several implications for the future.

There may be a need to ensure that national policies are more closely linked to available evidence. For example, there is little high-quality evidence that community matrons reduce hospitalizations, even though all regions are required to employ them. Better national guidance on the most effective approaches are needed in order to reduce variation in care, ensure care is more evidence based, and improve equity of access. Furthermore, the role of policy initiatives must be clearer. Policy-makers and service providers need to consider the degree to which policies focus on cost saving or improvement of health and quality of life.

PCTs have a great deal of autonomy over how they spend their budget. This means that a national business case may be needed for implementing the NHS Health and Social Care Model locally. Local service commissioners and chief executives may be most concerned with "breaking even" and would therefore need to know which initiatives are cost-effective in the short term. There is a need for a national approach to evaluation, looking at the different models, learning from the results, and making necessary improvements. Adequate time is needed to test the impact of new services and policies, rather than making constant changes. There may also be a need for more appropriate measures of success. Reducing emergency admissions, which is a high national priority, may be a poor indicator of good chronic disease management because of the multiple causes of admission. Developing better information support and decision systems may be crucial to ongoing evaluation and service improvement. This includes the capacity to share information between providers, and increasing confidence of providers and policy-makers to interpret and apply data. Potentially conflicting incentives should be avoided, for example, the inconsistency between policies such as "Payment by Results" and the creation of Foundation Hospitals compared to the goals set out in *Our health, our care, our say* (Department of Health 2006a). Finally, there appears to be good evidence to support self-care initiatives. There is a case for considering how these strategies could be further rolled out in England, with active support for providers.

The NHS Health and Social Care Model was initiated relatively recently and is likely to provide the general vision for the near future. Although the initial focus has been centred around case management, it is recognized that all components of the model need to be implemented and incentivized. Much of the planned future direction is reflected in the commitments set out in the policy document *Our health, our care, our say*, which emphasizes the need to:

- empower people with long-term conditions to do more to care for themselves by giving them better access to information and personalized care plans;
- better support informal carers, including short-term respite and training;
- increase investment in training and development of skills for staff who care for people with ongoing needs;
- improve collaboration between health and social care services to create multidisciplinary networks that support people with the most complex needs.

The main focus is on managing people with complex needs in order to minimize their use of services, moving care from hospitals into community or primary care settings. In principle, there is an ongoing commitment to chronic disease management by:

- investing in staff (specifically through new roles, ongoing training and competency frameworks, encouragement of multidisciplinary working, providing toolkits and workforce development programmes, as well as contracts for GPs and pharmacists with built-in incentives and recruitment drives to attract a broad range of staff);
- supporting innovation by setting up groups to test new models and by publicizing the findings of local and international evidence;
- developing information systems through planned national information sharing approaches and joint social care and health performance management frameworks;
- highlighting the importance of supported self-management and the role of service users in planning, implementing and evaluating services through the Expert Patients Programme, Patient and Public Involvement Forums, and trials of "individual budgets" where service users control spending.

While the approach taken in England may be sustainable in general terms (Table 3.2), there is less certainty that it will be successful in managing and minimizing the burden of chronic conditions. This is because there has been little evaluation of the NHS Health and Social Care Model and the premise(s) upon which it is based. Furthermore, while the policies may be laudable and individual components may have some benefits, the extent to which the overall vision is being implemented in practice is unclear, as is the level of ongoing evaluation.

Table 3.2 Chronic disease management in England: strengths and weaknesses

	Strengths	Weaknesses	Opportunities	Threats
Policy content	Focus on self-care Focus on care in the community Based on consultative process	Conflicting policies and incentives Budgets devolved to small areas	Opportunity to incentivize changes within acute sector Opportunities to build on local planning and SWOT analysis	Lack of ongoing national evaluation Lack of focus on equitable access
Policy consistency	Attempts to provide joint policy for health and social care	Some potentially competing policies Lack of legal requirements to build on model	Possibility of nationally recognized business case for chronic care	Varying local interpretation Competing policies may polarize primary and secondary care
Short- versus long-term perspective	Mix of long-term aims and short-term goals	Expectation of large scale reductions in admissions within short time frame	Flexibility to change as new evidence emerges	Lack of time and resource allocated to examining impacts Too great a focus on quick wins
Influence of electoral cycles (change in government)	Potential for voters to influence where spending is directed	Policy is greatly influenced by electoral cycles	Potentially inconsistent or problematic policies can be reversed	Lack of continuation and consistency Uncertainty for staff

(cont.)

Table 3.2 *(cont.)*

	Strengths	Weaknesses	Opportunities	Threats
Impact of institutional framework	Includes control at local level so decisions can be based on local needs	May be insufficient resourcing at local level to implement national policies	Mix of local, regional and national organizations to provide support	Lack of continuation and consistency Uncertainty for staff Regular changes in organizational configuration
Impact of macroeconomic conditions / constraints	Greater health spending in recent years, some of which has targeted disease management	Large focus on debt reduction and cost recovery rather than on improving well-being	Practice-based commissioning policies may be influenced by local needs	Devolved control of budgets may lead to inequitable service provision
Influence of other agencies / policies (e.g. WHO, European Commission)	International evidence considered when developing national policies	Evidence is sometimes considered after policies are implemented (e.g. case managers)	Opportunities to learn from other countries and trial new models, as well as sharing local experiences	Localized control may lead to being insular and less aware of international trends

Source: Authors' own compilation.

Notes: WHO: World Health Organization; SWOT: Strengths, weaknesses, opportunities and threats.

References

Billings J et al. (2006). *Case finding algorithms for patients at risk of re-hospitalisation. PARR1 and PARR2.* London, King's Fund, Health Dialog Analytic Solutions, New York University Center for Health and Public Service Research.

Boaden R et al. (2005). *Evercare evaluation interim report: implications for supporting people with long-term conditions.* Manchester, National Primary Care Research and Development Centre.

Boaden R et al. (2006). *Evercare evaluation: final report.* Manchester, National Primary Care Research and Development Centre.

Bower P et al. (2006). Recruitment to a trial of self-care skills training in long-term health conditions: analysis of the impact of patient attitudes and preferences. *Contemporary Clinical Trials,* 27:49–56.

British Medical Association & NHS Employers (2006). *Revisions to the GMS contract 2006/07.* London, NHS Employers, British Medical Association.

Care Services Improvement Partnership (2006) [web site]. Welcome to the Individual Budgets Pilot Programme web site. London, Departement of Health Policy and Innovation Division (http://individualbudgets.csip.org.uk/index.jsp, accessed 13 August 2008).

Department of Health (2001). *National service framework for diabetes: standards.* London, Department of Health.

Department of Health (2003). *Delivering investment in general practice: implementing the new GMS contract.* London, Department of Health.

Department of Health (2004a). *Practice-based commissioning. Engaging practices in commissioning.* London, Department of Health.

Department of Health (2004b). *The NHS Improvement Plan.* London, Department of Health.

Department of Health (2004c). *Chronic disease management: A compendium of information.* London, Department of Health.

Department of Health (2005a). *Supporting people with long-term conditions. An NHS and social care model to support local innovation and integration.* London, The Stationery Office.

Department of Health (2005b). *Supporting people with long-term conditions: Liberating the talents of nurses who care for people with long-term conditions.* London, Department of health.

Department of Health (2005c). *Self care – A real choice: Self care support – A practical option.* London, Department of Health.

Department of Health (2006a). *Our health, our care, our say: a new direction for community services*. London, The Stationery Office.

Department of Health (2006b). *Making it happen: pilots, early implementers and demonstration sites. Health and social care working together in partnership*. London, Department of Health (http://www.diabetes.nhs.uk/downloads/making_it_happen_pilots_early_implementers_and_demo_sites.pdf, accessed 13 August 2008).

Department of Health (2006c). *Caring for people with long-term conditions: An education framework for community matrons and case managers*. London, Department of Health.

Department of Health (2006d). *Independent sector treatment centres*. London, Department of Health (Report from Ken Anderson, Commercial Director, department of health to the Secretary of State for Health).

Department of Health (2006e). R&D annual reports by NHS organizations in England for 2006 [online database]. London, Department of Health (http://www.nrr.nhs.uk/default.htm, accessed 13 August 2008).

Department of Health (2007). *Commissioning framework for health and well-being*. London, Department of Health.

Downing A et al. (2007). Do the UK Government's new Quality and Outcomes Framework (QOF) scores adequately measure primary care performance? A cross-sectional survey of routine health care data. *BioMed Central Health Services Research,* 17:166.

EPPCIC (2007) [web site]. About Expert Patients. Greater London, Expert Patients Programme Community Interest Company (http://www.expertpatients.co.uk/public/default.aspx, accessed 13 August 2008).

Gravelle et al. (2007). Impact of case management (Evercare) on frail elderly patients: controlled before and after analysis of quantitative outcome data. *British Medical Journal,* 334:31.

Ham C et al. (2006). *Making the shift: interim evaluation report*. Birmingham, University of Birmingham Health Services Management Centre.

HM Treasury (2004). *2004 spending review. New public spending plans 2005–2008*. London, HM Treasury.

Hutt R, Rosen R, McCauley J (2004). *Case managing long-term conditions. What impact does it have in the treatment of older people?* London, King's Fund.

ISIP (2007). The principles of integrated service transformation [web site]. Integrated Service Transformation Programme. London, Department of

Health Integrated Service Transformation Programme (http://www.isip.nhs.uk/, accessed 13 August 2008).

Khunti K et al. (2007). Quality of diabetes care in the UK: comparison of published quality-of-care reports with results of the Quality and Outcomes Framework for Diabetes. *Diabetic Medicine,* 24:1436–1441.

National Collaborating Centre for Chronic Conditions (2007) [web site]. National Collaborating Centre for Chronic Conditions. London, Royal College of Physicians (http://www.rcplondon.ac.uk/college/ncc-cc/, accessed 13 August 2008).

NICE (2007) [web site]. National Institute for Health and Clinical Excellence. London, National Institute for Health and Clinical Excellence (http://www.nice.org.uk/, accessed 13 August 2008).

NPCRDC (2005). *NPCRDC briefing paper: How has the Expert Patients Programme been delivered and accepted in the NHS during the pilot phase?* Manchester, National Primary Care Research and Development Centre (http://www.npcrdc.ac.uk/Publications/EPP_briefing_paper.pdf, accessed 13 August 2008).

NHS Employers (2006a). *Improving services for people with long-term conditions through large-scale workforce change.* London, NHS Employers.

NHS Employers (2006b) [web site]. Agenda for change at a glance. (http://www.nhsemployers.org/pay-conditions/pay-conditions-198.cfm, accessed 13 August 2008).

NHS Institute for Innovation and Improvement (2007) [web site]. NHS Institute for Innovation and Improvement. Warwick, NHS Institute for Innovation and Improvement (http://www.institute.nhs.uk/, accessed 13 August 2008).

NHS Modernisation Agency and Skills for Health (2005). *Case management competences framework for the care of people with long-term conditions.* Bristol, NHS Modernisation Agency and Skills for Health.

NHS National Workforce Projects (2006). *Long-term conditions: Workforce development resource pack.* Manchester, NHS National Workforce Projects.

NHS Networks (2007) [web site]. NHS Networks. London, NHS Networks (http://www.networks.nhs.uk/1.php, accessed 13 August 2008).

Parker H (2006). *Making the shift: a review of NHS experience.* Birmingham, University of Birmingham and NHS Institute for Innovation and Improvement.

Singh D (2005a). *Transforming chronic care: Evidence about improving care for people with long-term conditions*. Birmingham, University of Birmingham and Surrey and Sussex PCT Alliance.

Singh D (2005b). *Which staff improve care for people with long-term conditions? A rapid review of the literature*. Birmingham, NHS Modernisation Agency and University of Birmingham.

Singh D (2006). *Making the shift: key success factors*. Birmingham, University of Birmingham and NHS Institute for Innovation and Improvement.

Singh D, Ham C (2006). *Improving care for people with long-term conditions: a review of UK and international frameworks*. Birmingham, University of Birmingham and NHS Institute for Innovation and Improvement.

Skills for Health (2008) [web site]. Skills for Health. Better skills, better jobs, better health. Bristol, Skills for Health (http://www.skillsforhealth.org.uk/, accessed May 2008).

Smith C et al. (2008). The impact of the 2004 NICE guideline and 2003 General Medical Services contract on COPD in primary care in the UK. *Quarterly Journal of Medicine,* 101:145–153.

South Yorkshire Academy for Health and Care Improvement (2006). *Reporting the effectiveness of community matrons – Doncaster*. Doncaster, South Yorkshire Academy for Health and Care Improvement.

The Information Centre for Health and Social Care (2007) [web site]. The Quality and Outcomes Framework 2006/07. London, The Information Centre for Health and Social Care (http://www.qof.ic.nhs.uk/, accessed 13 August 2008).

Chapter 4
France

Isabelle Durand-Zaleski, Olivier Obrecht

Context

The French health care system is mainly funded through health insurance under the supervision of the State. Since 1945, health care coverage has gradually expanded and with the 2000 Universal Health Coverage Act (CMU) all legal residents of France are now covered by the public Social Health Insurance (SHI) system. The SHI is mandatory and covers approximately 75% of total health expenditure. At the time of writing 92% of the population have complementary voluntary health insurance to offset statutory co-payments that are common for goods or services (Allonier et al. 2006).

Since 1996, national expenditure levels for health insurance are defined annually by law (Social Security Funding Act (SSFA)), supported by a government report describing the future direction of national health policy. The 1996 reform also reinforced the role of the country's regions, creating 22 regional hospital authorities (Agences régionales d'hospitalisation, ARH) and the Regional Unions of Insurance Funds (URCAM) (Sandier et al. 2004).

The Government determines health policies, the principles of which have been endorsed by Parliament, including a specific law on public health adopted in 2004. The State is also responsible for safety within the health system, with several agencies having been created since 1991 to oversee safety measures (for example, blood supply, medical products (including pharmaceuticals) and services, food products).

The delivery of health services is by public and private providers, covering both ambulatory and hospital care. Fee-for-service payments remain the general system for remunerating services in ambulatory care. The SHI annually agrees fees with the relevant professional unions representing the ambulatory care sector. The hospital sector is overseen by the ARHs, which allocate funding to individual hospitals (since 2005 based on a payment-per-case system) and define the level of service provision necessary to cover the needs of the population in a given region. Specifically, ARHs are responsible for the planning of resources and capacity of hospital care. However, since ARH directors are appointed by the Council of Ministers and are directly responsible to the Minister of Health, the planning process remains largely under the control of the executive. Among other things, ARHs determine the number and size of hospitals, the volume of certain types of services, and the quantity and allocation of expensive technology.

Regional planning is further specified in the Regional Strategic Health Plan (SROS), which sets out the development goals for regional provision over a 5-year period according to national or regional priorities. For example, each region has defined priority areas for service delivery, such as palliative care, suicide, cardiovascular diseases and chronic renal failure. The main aim of the SROS is to promote networks of hospitals within a region in which each hospital provides care according to its technical capacity.

This is further supported by the URCAMs, which coordinate the work of the three major social health insurance (SHI) schemes at the regional level and which work with the ARHs to encourage the creation of provider networks.

One of the key concerns in the French health care system has been a perceived lack of coordination and continuity of care, both at the ambulatory level and between ambulatory and hospital care. Several recent developments have aimed to address this weakness. These include the aforementioned 1996 reform, which introduced mechanisms to stimulate pilot projects using different provider networks at the local level and the 2001 SSFA, which provided for an extension for five years of provider networks projects. The subsequent 2002 SSFA introduced specific budgets for these projects. The 2002 Patients' Rights and Quality of Care Act brought together all initiatives under the health network concept, also introducing the formal designation of the "health network". It aims to strengthen the coordination, continuity and interdisciplinarity of health care provision, with a focus on selected population groups, disorders or activities.

Two other important steps in addressing the challenge of chronic disease have been the Public Health Law mentioned earlier and the Health Insurance Reform Act, both passed in 2004. The Public Health Law defines five major health plans and 104 public health priorities with individual target indicators for the period 2005–2009. The targets are organized into 22 categories, of which 11 concern chronic conditions or diseases. Alongside four major health plans, targeting cancer, rare diseases, health and environment and unhealthy behaviour, the Law also foresaw the development of a (fifth) national public health plan for people with chronic illness, which was published in 2007 (Ministère de la Santé et des Solidarités 2007).

The Health Insurance Reform Act reformed the regulation and financing of health care and has introduced a reform of the ALD procedure, as described later.

Analysing the response

Approaches to chronic disease management

In France, there are two major approaches to chronic disease management: the long-term disease (ALD) procedure and the health network approach; this section examines these two approaches in turn.

The French long-term disease (ALD) procedure

One key feature of the French social insurance system is the principle of patient co-payments for goods and services, which has been in place since the inception of the system in 1945. However, exemptions from co-payments exist for those whose health care costs could exceed their ability to pay, in the form of the ALD procedure, which targets those with long-term conditions.

The ALD procedure, as defined by the SHI, comprises a list of 30 (mostly chronic) diseases or disease groups. All expenses related to the treatment of one of the ALD diseases will be covered fully by the public system. Eligibility for exemption from co-payments for a patient with any of these conditions is determined by the GP presenting the patient's details to the health insurance, which in turn will decide whether or not the patient qualifies for full coverage. Patients with multiple conditions or with a (costly) single condition not listed (for example, a rare disease) may also be eligible for full coverage under the ALD system, if accepted by the relevant health insurance fund.

In recent years, the addition of new conditions to the ALD list was determined for the most part by the level of costs associated with treatment of the condition, that is, the condition was added as soon as a new costly treatment became available (for example human immunodeficiency virus (HIV), hepatitis, multiple sclerosis). As a result, the ALD list comprises all the main chronic conditions, although not all disease stages are always considered (for example depression and COPD will be considered only if at an advanced stage) (Table 4.1).

Table 4.1 *List of long-term disease (ALD) conditions*

No.	Disease/disease group	No.	Disease/disease group
1	Disabling stroke	16	Parkinson's disease
2	Aplastic anaemia and other chronic cytopenias	17	Hereditary metabolic conditions requiring long-term specialized treatment
3	Chronic arteriopathies with ischaemic manifestations	18	Cystic fibrosis
4	Complex schistosomiasis	19	Chronic nephropathy and primary nephrotic syndrome
5	Severe heart failure, arrythmias, valvular cardiomyopathy, congenital cardiomyopathy	20	Paraplegia
6	Active chronic diseases of the liver and cirrhoses	21	Polyarteritis nodosa, acute disseminated erythematous lupus, generalized progressive scleroderma
7	Primary severe immunodeficiency requiring long-term treatment, infection by HIV virus	22	Severe evolutive rheumatoid polyarthritis
8	Diabetes type 1, diabetes type 2	23	Long-term psychiatric conditions
9	Severe forms of neurological and muscular conditions (of which myopathy), serious epilepsy	24	Ulcerative colitis and evolutive Crohn's disease
10	Chronic severe constitutional and acquired haemoglobinopathies, haemolysis	25	Multiple sclerosis
11	Haemophilia and constitutional conditions of severe haemostasis	26	Evolutive structural scoliosis (the angle of which is equal to or over 25 degrees) until rachidian maturation
12	Severe arterial hypertension	27	Severe ankylosing spondylarthritis
13	Coronary heart disease	28	Organ transplant sequelae
14	COPD	29	Active TB, leprosy
15	Alzheimer's disease and other dementias	30	Malignant tumours, malignant lymphatic or haematopoietic tissue

Source: L'Assurance Maladie en Ligne 2006.

Notes: ALD: Affections de longue durée (long-term disease/disorder); HIV: Human immunodeficiency virus; TB: Tuberculosis; COPD: Chronic obstructive pulmonary disease.

Until 2004, the ALD procedure served mainly as mechanism to protect patients with long-term illness from financial hardship associated with treatment. As such, it provides valuable information on the direct medical costs of major chronic diseases. However, the ALD procedure was not primarily intended to be a mechanism for disease management, even though it does identify and facilitate monitoring of individuals with chronic disease. Despite a relatively hands-on process of acceptance into the ALD system, until recently it did not provide for measures to accompany the patient through treatment and care. The role of the health insurance funds was limited to periodically assessing whether the patient remained eligible for ALD coverage and that fully reimbursed prescriptions are truly related to the declared disease(s).

This situation changed with the 2004 Health Insurance Reform Act which, against the background of high growth in the number of ALD beneficiaries, sought to thoroughly transform the overall care process by:

- improving the quality of care using specific care pathways and monitoring of patient information;
- sharing common guidelines between GPs, specialists and medical advisors for the main chronic diseases, and promoting continuous medical education in this area;
- reducing the financial burden caused by unnecessary examinations or treatments (while accepting a simultaneous rise of some costs related to previously inadequate treatment of some patients);
- defining more clearly – and thus reducing – expenses for services targeting chronic disease individually;
- strengthening the role of the primary care physician (or GP) (not only for ALD patients) within the French health care system.

In line with these objectives, every French insured citizen now has to present a referral letter by her/his GP when seeking specialist care. Failure to do so results in higher co-payments being incurred by the patient. The ALD procedure itself has been revised as follows.

- the referring GP is responsible for establishing a care protocol for each patient requiring ALD coverage.
- the care protocol must clearly define the patient's clinical pathway, the health professionals involved, the treatments prescribed, and the planned follow-up. Acceptance of the protocols remains under the control of the health insurance funds.
- protocols must be defined for each condition within the ALD system by the French National Authority for Health (HAS) (see later); and

- the GP must obtain signed consent from the patient regarding the care protocol and the patient must present the protocol to every specialist s/he visits in order to qualify for full reimbursement, otherwise s/he will have to pay the usual co-payment rate (25% on average).

GPs receive an annual fee of €40 per ALD patient, funded by the SHI, representing an annual total of approximately €300 million. However, other than establishing the care protocol, GPs are not specifically held accountable. It has been estimated that approximately 80% of people with diabetes in France are covered by the ALD procedure.

The health network approach

As noted previously, a main weakness of the French health care system has been a lack of coordination between providers and sectors. In response, new models of health care delivery were being piloted from 1999–2000. The aim was to bring together into a network the health professionals involved in the management of a given condition, and to provide patients with previously unavailable services (such as patient education and specialist foot care) by offering special payment mechanisms to service providers. The health network approach was formally established by the 1996 Ordinances (Social Security Reform Law) and formalized under the 2002 Patients' Rights and Quality of Care Act, which defined the overall objectives and general organization of the networks. However, type, scope and distribution of health networks vary considerably from one region to another. This section focuses on networks targeting diabetes; it draws largely on a 2006 report presented to the Minister of Health by the Audit Group of Health and Social Affairs (IGAS) (IGAS 2006).

In 2006 there were approximately 450 networks operating in France, of which approximately 80% target chronic conditions (including cancer and palliative care), but most focus on diabetes. As of September 2006, there were 69 networks for diabetic patients (with a total budget of €14.5 million), involving an estimated 14 000 health professionals providing care to approximately 44 000 patients. On average, each network manages the services for approximately 800 patients (Association Nationale de Coordination des Réseaux Diabète 2006).

Patients join a network through their physician (usually the GP) or directly. Once they have given informed consent, they may freely access all services provided by the network. These might include educational sessions, dietary counselling, supervised weight loss and exercise programmes. This is a major incentive for patients who would previously have had to pay for these services. Each patient benefits from an individualized care plan, coordinated with other networks if necessary.

Health networks involve a wide range of health care professionals. For example, diabetes networks bring together primary care physicians and specialists, nurses, dieticians, podiatrists, physical therapists, biologists and pharmacists. Diabetes networks have transferred education sessions and nutrition counselling services from the hospital to the ambulatory setting. This was made possible by a change in legislation, permitting dieticians to provide services outside the hospital and to invoice the SHI. These networks have also set up training sessions for primary care physicians, nurses and physiotherapists, coming under the responsibility of hospital physicians or office-based specialists. The role of nurses and dieticians has thus been enhanced by the creation of networks.

Diabetes networks have encouraged patient empowerment and self-management. Support for patient self-management is mostly in the form of information and training sessions, for example on foot care, insulin injections, diet and exercise. Patients are encouraged to enter into a contractual relationship with the network professionals. The basis of the contract is to achieve realistic therapeutic goals. For patients with diabetes, goals may include attainment of adequate HbA1c levels, weight reduction and smoking cessation. At the time of enrolment, patients with diabetes receive a diary and a monthly information letter (REVEDIAB 2007). They are offered an annual assessment of their needs, focused in particular on cardiovascular risk factors. For patients with additional needs (such as obesity and/or substance abuse), the diabetes network liaises with other specialized networks and provides access to those services.

Treatment is guided by evidence-based protocols on a range of interventions, such as dietary recommendations, management of cardiovascular risk factors, insulin treatment and foot care. Protocols set out the specific responsibilities of each professional within the network. Fig. 4.1 illustrates the care pathway for a patient receiving insulin therapy, also highlighting the services that are not available to patients outside the network. Computerized decision support is not yet in use, although projects are being piloted for patients with vascular disease.

A patient journey: France

Patients with chronic conditions are typically diagnosed by a GP. Here we describe a typical journey of a fictitious patient, a 54-year-old woman with type 2 diabetes and COPD. She has a leg ulcer and moderate retinopathy. The patient is also moderately obese (BMI of 27). She has been unemployed for three years, receives social assistance benefits, and lives on her own.

It is common and financially beneficial to the patient if her GP helps her to apply for the ALD procedure for diabetes and to complete a care protocol form, which will then be submitted to the local health insurance fund. As diabetes is

Fig. 4.1 *Follow-up protocol for insulin therapy*

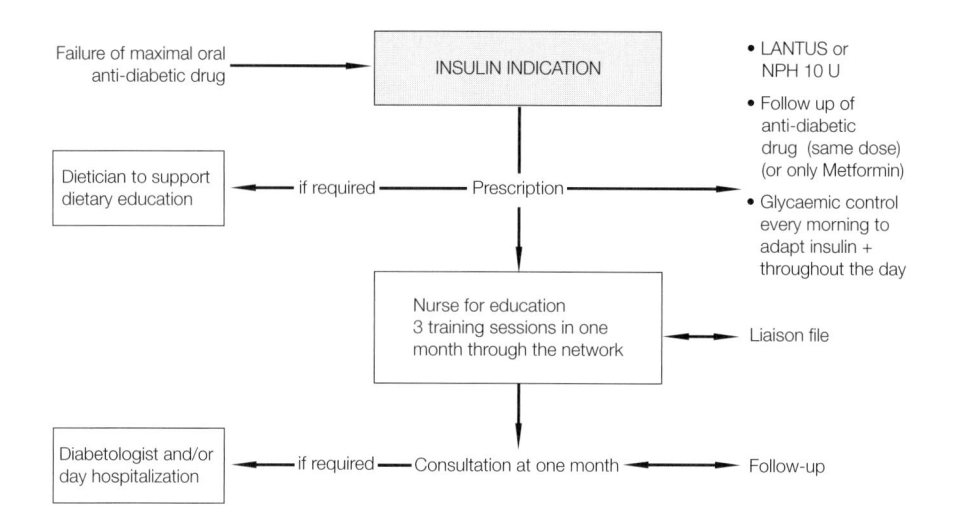

```
Failure of maximal oral ──────────▶ ┌──────────────────┐         • LANTUS or
  anti-diabetic drug                │ INSULIN INDICATION│           NPH 10 U
                                    └──────────────────┘
                                             │                   • Follow up of
                                             │                     anti-diabetic
┌──────────────────┐                         │                     drug (same dose)
│ Dietician to support│◀── if required ── Prescription ──────────▶  (or only Metformin)
│ dietary education│                         │
└──────────────────┘                         │                   • Glycaemic control
                                             │                     every morning to
                                             │                     adapt insulin +
                                             ▼                     throughout the day
                                  ┌──────────────────────┐
                                  │ Nurse for education  │
                                  │ 3 training sessions in one │◀── Liaison file
                                  │ month through the network  │
                                  └──────────────────────┘
                                             │
                                             ▼
┌──────────────────┐
│ Diabetologist and/or│◀── if required ── Consultation at one month ──▶ Follow-up
│ day hospitalization│
└──────────────────┘
```

Source: Adapted from REVEDIAB 2007.

currently a disease with no restrictions on acceptance under the ALD scheme, her application will be accepted. Once the diagnosis is established, the patient will automatically qualify for full ALD coverage if requested by the GP.

Once in the ALD system the patient will have at her disposal a full range of paid services, including specialist visits, medication, self-management support tools and, if necessary, hospitalization. Full coverage of costs is only granted for expenses related to the ALD condition; any other service or device (for example, dental prostheses) still requires co-payment.

As there is no structured, individualized disease management, it is the responsibility of the patient and her GP (along with specialists) to ensure her care pathway. The quality of care and coordination of multiple interventions depend on her relationship with the GP and the specialists. The 2004 reform set out to systematize this coordination, but concrete tools for implementation are not as yet in effect, except in the case of patients belonging to a health network.

Patients can join a network either via their physician (usually the GP) or directly (5%). Once they have given their informed consent and thereby formally enrolled in the network, they have free access to all services provided by the network. In addition, they may also access educational sessions, dietary counselling, supervised weight loss and exercise programmes, in partnership with another networks (for example, networks on weight control (such as ROMDES) (ROMDES 2006) and substance abuse (such as RAVMO) (RAVMO 2007)) (Fig. 4.2).

If patients cannot access health networks because they do not exist in their locality, one other option is the Maisons du diabète (diabetes homes) which are located in 20 cities throughout France (Association l'Union des Maisons du Diabète de la Nutrition et du Coeur 2007). These homes are non-profit-making institutions where diabetic patients have free access to nurses and dieticians for educational sessions. They also provide information leaflets on nutrition and other lifestyle issues. Both networks and diabetes homes cover approximately 5% of French diabetic patients.

Fig. 4.2 *Patient journey in a diabetes health network*

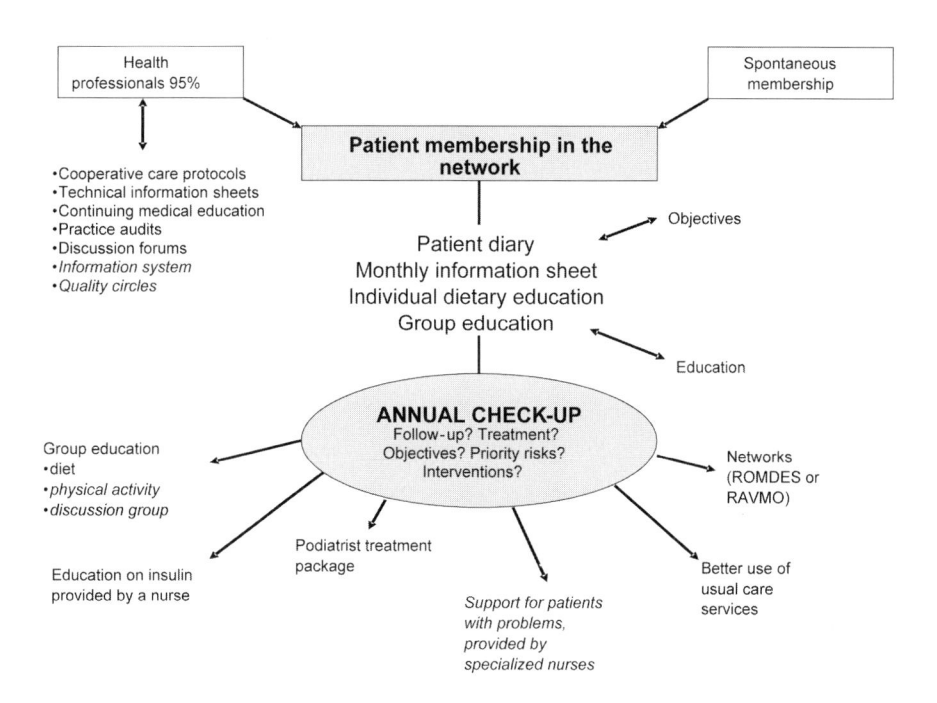

Source: Adapted from REVEDIAB 2007.

Notes: The services in italic are available as of 2004; ROMDES: Obesity network in the Essonne region; RAVMO: Substance abuse network in the Val-de-Marne Ouest region.

Health system features supporting programmes

Targets, standards and guidelines

The 2004 Health Insurance Reform Act, reforming the regulation and financing of health care in France, created a new public scientific body, the aforementioned French National Authority for Health (HAS). The HAS is an independent body, tasked to assess procedures related to pharmaceuticals, medical devices and health care and to produce national guidelines. It plays a key role in the development of guidelines for treatment of chronic diseases and defining eligibility criteria for inclusion in the ALD system.

Thus, for each ALD, the HAS develops (1) medical criteria of eligibility; (2) evidence-based operational protocols describing the clinical pathway for optimal management; and (3) a list of corresponding medical and allied services and products (eligible for full coverage under the ALD system). These are developed by a working group comprised of experts in the relevant field, GPs and patients' representatives, and are subsequently validated after field testing for relevance, feasibility and acceptability by all categories of users. The HAS also estimates patients' residual average out-of-pocket expenses.

There is an expectation that the production of updated protocols and recommendations should be integrated with three other important changes under way to optimize chronic disease management in France: (1) the development of an electronic personal medical record; (2) increased patient responsibility for health care (self-management); and (3) a mandatory role for GPs as key coordinators of individualized health care.

In addition, in 2006 a special agreement was signed between the SHI and unions representing medical doctors regarding follow-up for diabetic patients. The agreement involves an annual assessment of patients' clinical pathways with the application of four quality indicators to be collected by GPs. This can be seen as a first step towards a "true" disease management process, involving both the SHI and referral doctors.

Health care workforce and capacity

In France, job descriptions of health care professions are legally defined. Thus, transferring competencies from one group of professionals to another requires changes in the corresponding law, as has been done on a pilot basis to transfer responsibility for diabetes education and counselling from endocrinologists to dieticians (Berland & Bourgueil 2006). An initial dietary prescription is the responsibility of the physician, while the follow-up is then performed by a dietician. Other pilots concern a range of other chronic or acute conditions using, for example, hospital nurses for follow-up for patients with end-stage renal disease and hepatitis C. Their task also includes ordering tests and revising pharmaceutical prescriptions. An evaluation of these pilots under the responsibility of the HAS, published in April 2008, recommended that the Government ensures the sustainability of the pilots before engaging in the major reshuffle required by the transfer to develop the appropriate education, legal and financial mechanism(s) (HAS 2008).

While it is too early to draw general conclusions from these pilots (and their scope is limited), some features are noteworthy. The general task of redefining health professionals' roles in France is difficult because of obstacles at different levels: beyond the legal barriers mentioned earlier, there are cultural and social barriers resulting in part from the financing mechanisms in place for physicians and nurses in private practice. Both professions are remunerated through a fee-for-service system, as opposed to being salaried. However, dieticians are usually salaried and work in hospitals, and there is no reimbursement for dietary education outside hospitals. Thus, nurses' unions tend to be reluctant about such transfer of competence for at least two stated reasons: first, that it might create a two-tiered profession; and second, that it would place nurses in a position subordinate to physicians, should the system be expanded to include private nurses (instead of hospital nurses only). Moreover, there are concerns about the specific training necessary for nurses who would take over new tasks, as well as the current lack of both nurses and physicians in rural areas.

Financial management and incentives

Between 2000 and 2005, the SHI invested roughly €650 million into health networks. This has been carried out through (1) the Fund for the Quality Improvement of Ambulatory Care (FAQVS) and, as of 2002, (2) the National and Regional Fund for the Development of Networks (DNDR (national) or DRDR (regional)). Both funds may be used to finance networks (infrastructure and operating costs), while the DNDR can also finance new services, as outlined earlier. Of a total of €650 million set aside, €500 million have been spent so far (Box 4.1). In addition to these funds, the SHI has spent €240 million for primary care physicians to coordinate the care of patients with chronic diseases, corresponding to a payment of €40 per patient suffering with an ALD.

In addition to a budget for infrastructure and operating costs, the SHI provides incentives to providers, involving set fees for individual yearly assessment (€50), foot care (€141), education (€100) and dietary counselling by nurses and dieticians (€70). These services are provided by nearly all networks and financed from the DRDR budget. The fees are paid for by the network in

> **Box 4.1 Costing patient care in health networks**
>
> The total cost per patient of being cared for by a network varies between €130 and €1000 (in addition to the usual medical costs). For example, a network for diabetic patients in the Provence region (RESDIAB) underwent a full financial (although preliminary) audit which estimated the annual cost per patient at an additional €1363, compared to diabetic patients outside the network. However, an audit of networks for elderly individuals financed by the SHI fund for agricultural workers concluded that the additional costs of the networks were offset by reduced hospital costs. There is a general agreement that the networks are to be considered as an investment in the future, rather than as a cost-saving tool. Decision-makers both in the Ministry of Health and the SHI have emphasized health promotion over cost–containment, requesting that networks document how additional expenditure has improved the health of patients.

addition to any other services claimed from the SHI by professionals, thus creating substantial financial incentives for providers who could not previously invoice the SHI for such services, typically those who work in private practice. All types of professionals can benefit from this incentive system, provided they sign the contractual agreement between the network and the SHI.

Non-financial incentives are implicit in the networks' definition and include preferential access to specialists with otherwise long waiting lists (such as ophthalmologists), access to continuing medical education and training programmes, and newsletters for patients containing dietary and other practical information. There are also negative incentives for providers, for example time commitment, fear of "losing" patients to other specialists and weakening of professional identity.

Evaluation and lessons learned

There is no single system to evaluate the management of chronic conditions in France. Health networks receiving public funding must by law undergo an annual internal quality audit and an external quality audit every three years. The audit includes an evaluation of all aspects of the network, including its structure, processes of care and, to a certain extent, the outcomes of services provided. The regional health authority that finances networks may act upon the results of these evaluations to either continue or discontinue budgets. However, for the majority of patients (that is, those not belonging to a network), no formal system exists.

The management of chronic disease in France has until very recently mainly depended on the initiative of health professionals, who chose whether or not to follow guidelines and coordinate their activities to provide comprehensive treatment. A failure to do so brought no financial penalties for patients who benefited from 100% coverage, regardless of the quality and quantity of prescriptions. In its 2006 report, the advisory group in charge of auditing the SHI (the "Haut Conseil pour l'Avenir de l'Assurance Maladie", the advisory group for the future of health insurance) highlighted the aforementioned lack of coordination between health professionals (Haut Conseil pour l'Avenir de l'Assurance Maladie 2006). Coordination may be improved with the strengthening of the primary care physician's gatekeeper role, but for a patient with a chronic disease, direct access to specialized care is permitted and does not result in any financial penalty.

An important element of the 2004 Health Insurance Reform Act was provision for an electronic patient record, expected to limit the duplication of prescriptions and to allow better coordination between health professionals for patients who require frequent health care. This computerized record is currently being tested at regional level but results are not yet available. Audits of networks that invested in the development of information systems in general found computerized health records not to be cost-efficient (Box 4.2). At the time of writing, most networks operate with a web site, but without computerized health records.

Box 4.2 National audit of health networks

In 2006 the Ministry of Health commissioned a national audit of networks in operation at that time. In general terms, the audit report remarked on the overall inefficiency of networks. While the efforts of health professionals who endeavoured to reduce inequalities in access to care and to introduce new preventive services were commended, the main criticism was directed at the main financing institutions (both the State and Social Health Insurance (SHI), in that neither acted upon the findings of internal audits of networks or requested more in-depth evaluations. The audit also noted that multi-professional networks did not substantially improve coordination of care between office- and hospital-based physicians and health professionals. New management tools, such as electronic medical records and decision support systems were found to be unsustainable: over €30 million had been invested into information systems but with only limited results, and this failure was mostly due to technical problems. Overall, networks were rated not to be very cost-efficient. The one positive aspect was the emerging willingness to tackle the issues of health care provision at regional level.

The Ministry of Health's Health and Social Affairs Audit Group (IGAS) carried out a thorough review of two networks which have been rated effective for patients and professionals, namely the diabetes and geriatric care networks. Thus, the diabetes networks were found to lead to improved adherence to national guidelines and clinical outcomes, such as improved HbA1C levels and weight loss. While geriatric care networks were found to be more heterogeneous than diabetes networks in that they do not share common care processes and guidelines, formal evaluations pointed to fewer pharmaceuticals prescriptions, fewer hospitalizations and lower mortality rate compared to a control group. Economic evaluations of geriatric networks indicated a possible breakeven: the cost saving from reduced prescriptions and hospital stays was offset by the additional network services costs (approximately €1000 per patient). However, the evaluations were limited in scope and cannot be generalized.

Networks have high fixed costs and must therefore attract a greater number of patients; at the moment only a small proportion (an estimated 0.5%) of the 8 million patients currently registered in the ALD system belong to a network. The success of networks is greatly dependent on professionals who promote those networks and on the availability of additional services provided free of charge.

However, in spite of the shortcomings elucidated earlier, there is a general perception that the programme of networks should be continued and a unified, central decision-making process promoted. This includes merging the existing financing mechanisms under one single fund, defining strategic priorities for networks at national level, consolidating evaluation processes with a set of common indicators mandated for all networks and implementing systematic financial audits. Medical evaluations and financial audits provided to both the SHI and the Ministry of Health should be used to inform decisions on resource allocation.

Investing in the future

Chronic disease management and patients' quality of life were identified as one of the top five priorities for the French public health policy in 2004 and, in 2005, the Ministry of Health's IGAS group carried out a comparative analysis of disease management models in the United States, Germany and the United Kingdom to identify lessons from their respective experiences that could be applied in France (Bras, Duhamel & Grass 2006).

At the time of writing, some components of the Chronic Care Model (CCM), as developed by Wagner (1998) are integrated into the French system (Box 4.3) with official support, yet many characteristics of the French health care system are likely to hinder the adoption of the entire model.

Box 4.3 Components of the Chronic Care Model in the French system

- Mobilize community resources to meet the needs of patients.
- Create a culture, organization and mechanisms that promote safe, high-quality care (including care coordination and incentives based on quality).
- Empower and prepare patients to manage their health and health care.
- Ensure the delivery of effective, efficient clinical care and self-management support (including task sharing among professionals and case management for patients with complex conditions).
- Promote clinical care, consistent with scientific evidence and patient preferences.
- Organize clinical information systems with patient and population data to facilitate care planning, information sharing and performance monitoring.

A major constraint remains the continued lack of coordination between medical and social services, despite several efforts within networks. This is largely due to the division of budgets and employees between the regions, the State and the SHI. Guidelines are produced at national level to ensure equal quality of care throughout the country. At the same time, however, the social services budgets and employees are the responsibility of regions and municipalities, and health professionals operate either in private practice or are salaried by the SHI. There is therefore no consistency either in authority or in resource allocation. As for the split funding of networks, the 2007 SSFA has unified the two funds into a single fund aimed at Quality and Coordination of Care, which is jointly controlled by the Government and the health insurance funds. This has opened up the possibility of better coordination of care policies.

While national guidelines on long-term conditions have been developed since the mid-1990s by the HAS (and its predecessor ANAES (French National Agency for Evaluation and Accreditation in Health)) in collaboration with health professionals, their integration into processes of care has met with resistance by some health professionals, and the exclusion of patient groups from the mainstream health care system has exacerbated the poor adoption of guidelines. Under the reformed ALD procedure, personalized care and follow-up protocols for patients with chronic disease are to be designed by the GP and agreed by the patient. However, whether these guidelines are being adequately understood and implemented is unclear because they have not yet been evaluated, despite the mandatory evaluation of GPs since 2004.

Furthermore, the 2004 Health Insurance Reform Act intended to reinforce the role of primary care physicians in coordinating care by introducing a gatekeeping function so as to optimize care in a cost-efficient way. Whether the reform will lead to the adoption of state-led managed care in France remains unclear (Rodwin & Le Pen 2004). However, it is doubtful that such a measure will have a significant impact, since more than 90% of patients already consult the same physician on a regular basis, but continue to experience difficulties in navigating through the system and benefiting from coordinated delivery of services.

The 2004 Health Insurance Reform Act also set out to enhance quality of care and to develop patient education, in order to improve self-management. While it is too soon to assess the commitment of GPs and the impact of the reform on health, it is noteworthy that health education programmes in France are scarce and not easily identified (Fournier et al. 2001).

While a wide range of measures has been introduced to enhance care for those with chronic disease(s), there has been little effort to synthesize these ostensibly disparate approaches into an overarching policy with defined objectives, implementation rules, incentives and enforcement mechanisms, jointly agreed or negotiated by key stakeholders. The mechanisms remain broadly doctor oriented and lacking the vital involvement of patients, despite ALD beneficiaries having to sign their care protocols (since this does not involve any real commitment).

What can be done to meet patients' needs in France better? The Ministry of Health's IGAS report (IGAS 2006) suggested two options. One emphasizes the primary care team, which comprises one or more physicians working closely and systematically with other health professionals to define precisely and to target common health outcomes for patients. The second option argues for specific interventions delivered by specially trained staff within disease management programmes as a complementary service to the usual care delivered by GPs. These programmes would be managed through call centres that would provide information, patient education and coaching, contributing to coordination of care and monitoring.

At the time of writing, DMPs seem to be the preferred option, at least in the short term. This is because – unlike countries where the primary care team is positioned as the central actor in the management of patient care – working conditions for doctors in France are not well suited to chronic disease management. Above and beyond the barriers to better chronic disease management described in this chapter, there continues to be strong cultural and professional reluctance to an intermediate type of chronic disease manager and to novel methods of monitoring health and delivering care.

At the same time, certain characteristics of the French health system are likely to promote the development and implementation of DMPs, as outlined in Table 4.2. Specifically, quality enhancement and cost reductions in hospital care are expected to be attainable. Also, although outpatient services and hospital information systems are not integrated, public insurers have access to information that will help identify patients with chronic disease and stratify them according to their level of risk, based on currently observed pathways. This will be further supported by the national uniform electronic medical record system which is currently being developed and tested. Finally, the 2007 national Public Health Plan on Quality of Life for the Chronically Ill (PQVMC) (Ministère de la Santé et des Solidarités 2007) promotes piloting (and financing of) DMPs, primarily targeting diabetes and heart failure, and in particular the development of education for diabetic patients. It will be the first attempt at chronic disease management in France that coherently and simultaneously involves health professionals, patients and the SHI system.

Table 4.2 *Chronic disease management in France: strengths and weaknesses*

Strengths	Weaknesses	Opportunities	Threats
Individual health care protocols for patients with long-term conditions became mandatory in 2005	Fragmentation of care	Growing patient demand for coordination and planned policy to respond to demand	Limited incentives for GPs to accept new responsibilities in the coordination of care
	Absence of adequate follow-up of individual protocols		
		A National Public Health Plan on Quality of Life for the Chronically Ill was published in 2007	Reluctance of professionals to engage in a payment system different from fee-for-service remuneration
Reinforced role of the primary care physician in the coordination of care	Lack of educational programmes and structures and of community resources		
	Lack of computerized medical data sharing		
Available guidelines for health professionals	Absence of adequate evaluation of practices	A planned development of patient therapeutic education and disease management programmes	Limited resources for patient education
A national list of defined chronic conditions			
		An electronic medical record currently under development	
		Doctors union engagement to develop disease management for diabetic patients (2006 Agreement signed with the SHI)	
		Mandatory evaluation of doctors' practices	

Source: Authors' own compilation.

Notes: SHI: Social Health Insurance; GP: General practitioner.

References

Allonier C, Dourgnon P, Rochereau T (2006). Health, health care and insurance survey 2004: First results. *IRDES Health Economics Letter,* 110:1–6.

Association l'Union des Maisons du Diabète de la Nutrition et du Coeur (2007) [web site]. Association l'Union des Maisons du Diabète de la Nutrition et du Coeur. Association l'Union des Maisons du Diabète de la Nutrition et du Cœur (http://www.maison-diabete.info/index.php, accessed 14 August 2008).

Association Nationale de Coordination des Réseaux Diabète (2006). Bilan d'activité des Réseaux Diabète – Octobre 2006. Montegron, Association Nationale de Coordination des Réseaux Diabète (http://www.asso-ancred.org/index.php?option=com_content&task=view&id=258&Itemid=163, accessed 21 May 2008).

Berland Y, Bourgueil Y (2006). *Cinq expérimentations de coopération et de délégation de tâches entre professions de santé.* Paris, Observatoire National de la Démographie des Professions de Santé.

Bras PL, Duhamel G, Grass E (2006). *Améliorer la prise en charge des maladies chroniques: les enseignements des experiences étrangères de «disease management».* Paris, Inspection Generale des Affaires Sociales (MoH).

Fournier C et al. (2001). Towards promotion, structuring and acknowledgement of patient education activities in France. *Patient Education and Counseling,* 44:29–34.

HAS (2008). *Délégation, transferts, nouveaux métiers… Comment favoriser des formes nouvelles de coopération entre professionnels de santé? Recommandation HAS en collaboration avec l'ONDPS.* Saint-Denis La Plaine Cedex, Haute Autorité de Santé.

Haut Conseil pour l'Avenir de l'Assurance Maladie (2006). *Rapport du Haut Conseil pour l'Avenir de l'Assurance Maladie.* Paris, Haut Conseil pour l'Avenir de l'Assurance Maladie.

IGAS (2006). *Contrôle et évaluation du fonds d'aide à la qualité des soins de ville (FAQSV) et de le dotation de développement des réseaux (DDR).* Paris, Inspection Generale des Affaires Sociales.

L'assurance Maladie en Ligne (2006). *Tableau I: Répartition du nombre d'ETM et taux d'incidence en fonction des 30 affections de la liste avec, pour chaque affection, la répartition en fonction du sexe et de l'âge moyen des bénéficiaires – Année 2006.* Paris, L'assurance Maladie en Ligne (http://www.ameli.fr/fileadmin/user_upload/documents/tableauI_2006.pdf, accessed 14 August 2008).

Ministère de la Santé et des Solidarités (2007). *Plan pour l'amélioration de la qualité de vie des personnes atteintes de maladies chroniques.* Paris, Ministère de la Santé et des Solidarités.

RAVMO (2007) [web site]. Réseau Addictions Val de Marne Ouest. Villejuif, Réseau Addictions Val de Marne Ouest (http://ravmo.org/, accessed 14 August 2008).

REVEDIAB (2007) [web site]. Réseau Expérimental Val de Marne Essonne de soins aux Diabétiques de type 2. Montegron, REVEDIAB (http://revediab.asso.free.fr/, accessed 14 August 2008).

Rodwin VG, Le Pen C (2004). Health care reform in France. The birth of state-led managed care. *New England Journal of Medicine*, 351:2259–2262.

ROMDES (2006) [web site]. Le réseau ROMDES. Ris Orangis, ROMDES (http://www.romdes.org/, accessed 14 August 2008).

Sandier S, Paris V, Polton D (2004). Health care systems in transition: France. *Health Systems in Transition*, 6(2):1–145.

Wagner E (1998). Chronic disease management: What will it take to improve care for chronic illness. *Effective Clinical Practice*, 1:2–4.

Chapter 5
Germany

Ulrich Siering

Context

In Germany, the main source of health care financing is statutory Social Health Insurance (SHI), which covers just under 90% of the population, while approximately 10% of the population has opted opt out of the statutory system and has complementary voluntary health insurance. Less than 1% of the population is without any coverage (Busse & Riesberg 2004). Coverage under the statutory SHI system is mandatory for employees whose gross income does not exceed a specified level; statutory SHI covers employees and their dependants as well as pensioners; and private insurance is purchased by those who are not required to join the statutory system, including civil servants and their dependants. Statutory SHI is financed through contributions from employers and employees (Busse & Riesberg 2004). The level of statutory SHI contributions is dependent on income, rather than individual risk, and is calculated as a proportion of income from gainful employment (or pensions) and benefits cover non-earning dependants without any surcharge.

Health care delivery is both public and private: ambulatory care is provided by office-based, private profit-making providers (family physicians and specialists), who usually run individual surgeries or small group practices. Patients are free to choose from among family physicians and specialists, except where patients have joined a "gatekeeper model" (*Hausarztmodell*) in which access to reimbursed care by specialist providers is available only following referral. Hospitals are owned and operated by a variety of public and private (non-profit-making or profit-making) organizations, providing only limited outpatient services; outpatient clinics or other institutions which employ physicians and primarily provide outpatient services are rare in Germany.

Ambulatory care is organized at the level of the federal states (*Länder*), through 17 regional physicians' associations (KVs). KVs are responsible for licensing SHI physicians and arranging reimbursement of services provided in the ambulatory sector. The reimbursement of inpatient services is carried out directly by health insurance funds.

Under the statutory SHI system, services are provided free at the point of access, although cost-sharing and co-payments are required, including a fee of €10 for the first contact with the family physician per quarter (and for consultations with other physicians without referral during the same quarter). The private insurance system is based on a cost-reimbursement principle: the patient is invoiced for the cost of medical services by the service provider, who is subsequently reimbursed by the respective private insurer.

The health care system in Germany operates on the principle of self-governance. The State is responsible for setting the legal framework, embodied in the Social Code Book V (SGB V), by which health insurance funds and service providers must abide. The most important body within the self-governing health system is the Federal Joint Committee (GBA), the highest decision-making body at federal level. It brings together the federal associations of sickness funds and the federal associations of provider groups (physicians, dentists and hospitals). It is responsible for defining the publicly financed package of services and setting quality standards for ambulatory, inpatient and intersectoral health care.

Since the 1990s the quality of the German health care system has been the subject of increasingly critical analysis. In 2001 the government-commissioned Advisory Council on the Assessment of Developments in the Health Care System (SVR) issued a report highlighting the dominance of acute care and the lack of prevention and rehabilitation; citing chronically ill patients as passive recipients of medical services; and highlighting inadequate training and information as well as the lack of participation by patients and their families (Sell 2005). The report identified inadequate use of scientific knowledge, the strict separation of the inpatient and ambulatory sectors, and a lack of incentives for the care of those with chronic disease as factors contributing to low quality of care. Disease management programmes (DMPs) were seen as a means to reduce deficits in the health care system, with Lauterbach et al. (2001) arguing that medical outcomes could be improved by greater use of evidence-based guidelines, structured care provision, the active involvement of patients and enhanced self-management. At the same time, there was an expectation that costs could be reduced by avoiding overprovision or inappropriate provision of services. In 2002 the Government formally introduced structured care, or disease management, programmes for those with chronic disease (DMPs) into the German health care system. Other strategies include provisions that enable selective contracting between sickness funds and providers to create more integrated models of care and the introduction of medical care centres (*Medizinische Versorgungszentren*), which provide care across several health care specialties (similar to the "polyclinic" model of care, a common feature of the health care system of the German Democratic Republic) (Ettelt et al. 2006). While acknowledging the importance of these and other approaches (for an overview see Hilfer, Riesberg & Egger (2007)), this chapter focuses on the German DMPs which have attracted considerable international attention.

Analysing the response

Approaches to chronic disease management

The legal framework for structured care programmes (or DMPs [2]) is set out in the SGB V. Defined as "*an organisational approach to medical care that involves the coordinated treatment and care of patients with chronic disease across boundaries between individual providers and on the basis of scientific and up-to-date evidence*" (Bundesversicherungsamt 2008), German DMPs are based on the following principles: treatment options should be based on the best available evidence; intersectoral care and treatment in specialized institutions should be promoted; patient self-management is an important component; and new quality assurance measures will be introduced.

The SGB V defines the areas of responsibility for the development of DMPs and has mandated the GBA to identify conditions suitable for DMPs and to develop and update regularly the content of DMPs. Criteria to be considered for DMPs include: a high number of (insured) individuals with the particular condition(s); potential for quality improvement; availability of evidence-based guidelines; requirement for an intersectoral approach to treatment; self-management influencing the course of the condition(s); and high costs related to the condition(s). The GBA subsequently identified the following conditions or groups of conditions as suitable for the development of a DMP: breast cancer; type 1 and 2 diabetes; coronary heart disease; and asthma and COPD. The first DMP, for breast cancer, was accredited in January 2003, followed in April of that year by the first DMP for type 2 diabetes, with coronary heart disease following in September 2004 and asthma and COPD in January 2006 (Fig. 5.1). It is important to note that individual regional activities to enhance care for those with chronic conditions had already been initiated before the formal introduction of DMPs. However, it was only with

---

2. The formal nomination, as set out in legislation, is "structured care programme for the chronically ill"; however, the term has been used synonymously with "disease management programmes" which, for simplicity, will also be used here.

Fig. 5.1 *Time line for the introduction of disease management programmes in Germany*

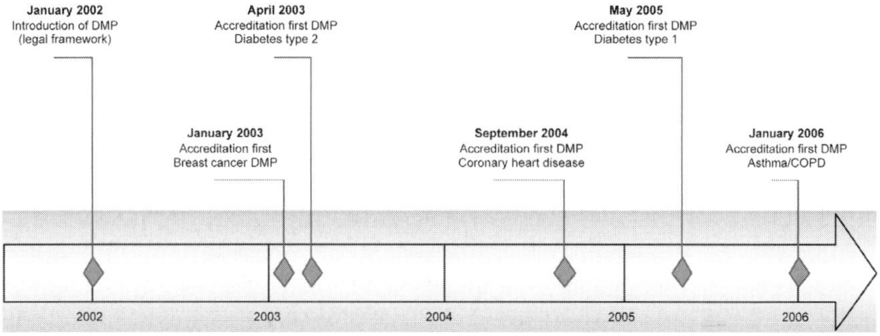

January 2002	Introduction of DMP (legal framework)
January 2003	Accreditation first Breast cancer DMP
April 2003	Accreditation first DMP Diabetes type 2
September 2004	Accreditation first DMP Coronary heart disease
May 2005	Accreditation first DMP Diabetes type 1
January 2006	Accreditation first DMP Asthma/COPD

Source: Adapted from Bundesministerium für Gesundheit 2006a.

Notes: DMP: disease management programme; COPD: Chronic obstructive pulmonary disease.

the 2002 amendments to the SGB V that DMPs for type 2 diabetes, breast cancer and coronary heart disease were introduced throughout the country.

Participation in DMPs is voluntary for both patients and providers. Participants can be either chronically ill patients with statutory SHI cover who meet certain medical conditions, or various service providers. Patients who wish to take part in a DMP have to choose a physician who coordinates their treatment within the DMP. This is usually the patient's family physician, who checks whether the patient meets the conditions for participation, as set out in the Regulation on Risk Structure Compensation (RSAV). The task of the family physician is then to carry out the ongoing coordination of care for the patient. This is further specified in the DMP, which sets out how and when specialists in private practice and hospitals should be involved in the patient's care alongside the family physician, so as to avoid gaps in care provision between the ambulatory and the inpatient sectors (see later).

Along with the general goal of improving the care of those with chronic conditions, individual DMPs have set disease-specific objectives. For example, the DMP for coronary heart disease is expected to reduce mortality, reduce the risk of developing heart attacks and cardiac failure, increase quality of life by minimizing suffering caused by angina pectoris, and maintain the patient's functional capacity.

Key components of any DMP, as stipulated in the regulations, include diagnosis; defining treatment goals; treatment planning; medical (such as pharmacological treatment) and nonmedical interventions (such as education, psychosocial support); patient education; rehabilitation; and intersectoral cooperation. To optimize cooperation between sectors involved in care provision, the regulatory framework has defined specific criteria for referral to secondary care if necessary, as illustrated in Table 5.1 for the diabetes DMP.

Table 5.1 *Criteria for coordinating care levels in the diabetes disease management programme*

Provider type	Tasks / Criteria for referral / admission
Coordinating family physician	• agreement on an individual treatment goal between physician and patient • adherence to care contents as stipulated by the RSAV • coordination of treatment • information, advising and registration of the patient • adherence to the quality targets of the DMP agreement • patient education • referral to and/or involvement of other specialists and psychotherapists • if applicable, referral to a hospital • drawing up of initial and follow-up documentation
Specialist or specialized institution	Complications requiring a referral to a specialist/practice/institution specializing in diabetes: • annual ophthalmological check-up • patients with retinopathy and proteinuria • failure to achieve target blood pressure within a maximum period of six months • failure to achieve the individually agreed HbA1c target value after a maximum of six months • (planned) pregnancy
Institution specialized in the treatment of diabetic foot	Presence of diabetic foot disease or high risk of ulceration
Hospital	• in case of emergency • in case of threatened metabolic crises • in case of serious specific metabolic crises • in case of an infected diabetic foot or acute neuro-osteopathic foot complications

Source: Adapted from Bundesministerium der Justiz 2008.

Notes: DMP: disease management programme; RSAV: Regulation on Risk Structure Compensation.

When participating in a DMP, physicians commit to take into consideration the main medical aspects of patient care, as set out in the regulations (Box 5.1). However, the guidelines for medical care are not binding, allowing the physician to deviate from them if the patient's situation justifies it, although in such cases the physician must inform the patient, for example, if medical products are used that are not specified in the regulations. Increasingly, however, physicians are expected to justify any deviation from the DMPs.

Patients who have registered with a DMP are expected to participate actively in the programme. Patients therefore undertake to adhere to planned appointments with their physician when registering. Failure to do so will result in having them to leave the programme. Patients are expected to participate in

Box 5.1 Formal development of disease management programmes in Germany

According to the Social Code Book V (SGB V), medical care within the disease management programmes (DMPs) should be drawn up on the basis of "the latest developments in medical science, while taking evidence-based guidelines into account". The legislation then defines the components to be addressed in the design of programmes: the conditions for the enrolment of insured individuals in a DMP; key points for treatment according to the latest developments in medical science; quality assurance and evaluation measures; training of services providers; training of insured participants; and uniform documentation.

The Federal Joint Committee (GBA) used a systematic procedure for drawing up the contents. The medical recommendations in the DMPs are based on a systematic review of the literature on core issues integral to the care of those with chronic disease(s) (see, for example, Kaiser, Krones & Sawicki (2003a), Kaiser, Krones & Sawicki (2003b), Kaiser, Jennen & Sawicki (2003)). In addition, the GBA uses consensus strategies and specialist evidence to formulate recommendations. Medical recommendations are supported by references to individual studies and/ or other publications in the formal description of each programme. Whether the requirements for organizational processes in the DMPs as set out in the legislation can actually be implemented in practice was not, however, systematically examined.

The key elements of medical treatment in the DMP, as developed by the GBA, are then be examined by the legislature and published in the Regulation on Risk Structure Compensation (RSAV)[1]. In addition, the RSAV defines specific organizational requirements for the implementation of the DMPs, as well as mandating the Federal Insurance Office to ensure adherence to RSAV provisions and the accreditation of DMPs (including reaccreditation after three years) (Gawlik 2005). The requirements set out in the RSAV apply to the entire statutory social health insurance (SHI) system.

---

1. The German RSAV, introduced in the 1990s, seeks to equalize differences among sickness funds related to contribution rates (arising from varying income levels within the insured population of a given fund) and to expenditure (arising from differences in the age and sex structure of the insured population).

the planning of treatment and if possible in formulating treatment goals, for example HbA1c target values in the DMP for type 2 diabetes. Each patient should, in principle, also have access to educational programmes specifically designed for their needs; classes are normally carried out in groups and are composed of four or five 90-minute sessions.

Patient education programmes must meet legally defined criteria: they must be systematic and targeted, and have been evaluated and published. Health insurance funds applying for accreditation must demonstrate that the proposed DMP provides an appropriate patient education programme or they may refer patients to an established programme already approved by the Federal Insurance Office (Bundesversicherungsamt 2005). Both physicians coordinating the programmes and health insurance funds are expected to encourage the active participation of patients; many funds provide information leaflets, and/or offer additional counselling or telephone hotlines.

Formal regulations explicitly address the psychological and psychosocial support of patients registered with a DMP, requesting the coordinating physicians to examine to what extent the underlying chronic disease(s) of the patient may benefit from psychotherapeutic or psychiatric treatment. However, the definition of psychological support remains vague in the DMP agreements concluded so far.

Distribution, uptake and coverage

DMPs are usually offered by all of the SHI funds in a given region. To set up a DMP, the health insurance fund will enter into a contract with the KV, which represents SHI doctors in private practice, alongside other actors such as the regional association of hospitals. Thus, all those with a chronic disease who are covered by the statutory system may join one or more programmes, if provided in the respective region.

By June 2006 there were approximately 250 SHI funds in Germany (Bundesministerium für Gesundheit 2006b). Each fund offers its own range of DMPs, which are available in a specific region, and as a consequence a high number of DMP contracts are concluded in Germany as a whole. For example, in June 2007 there were more than 14 000 DMPs (1952 for type 1 diabetes, 3325 for type 2 diabetes, 2846 for breast cancer and 3016 for coronary heart disease) (Bundesversicherungsamt 2008). This seemingly large number of programmes is deceptive, however, as their content and organizational structures are very similar. The high number of DMPs conceals the fact that normally all regional sickness funds only negotiate one DMP contract for one chronic condition with the regional association of SHI physicians. However, each SHI fund will have to apply individually for accreditation through the Federal Insurance Office. Programmes are usually complemented by some service add-ons that are specific to the fund, but which do not normally fundamentally alter the overall service arrangements within a given DMP. Differences between programmes for similar conditions are thus marginal and generally relate to certain patient benefits (such as telephone hotlines and partial reimbursement of insurance contributions).

As the number of DMPs increases, so does the number of patients registered within them. Thus, between October 2004 and December 2005 the number of patients that received care as part of a DMP doubled, from approximately 1 million to over 2 million (Bundesministerium für Gesundheit 2006c). However, there are few specific data on the proportion of patients with chronic conditions who are registered with DMPs. It has been estimated that 65–70% of those with type 2 diabetes are registered with a DMP (AOK Baden-Württemberg 2006, Nordrheinische Gemeinsame Einrichtung Disease-Management-Programme GbR 2006); however, there is no information on the proportion of patients registered with coronary heart disease, asthma and COPD DMPs.

As for physicians participating in DMPs, again there are no precise numbers as participation is not systematically recorded. However, it has been estimated that between 60% and 75% of family physicians who could take part in type 2 diabetes and coronary heart disease DMPs actually do so (Nordrheinische Gemeinsame Einrichtung Disease-Management-Programme GbR 2006).

A patient journey: Germany

Here we describe a patient journey for a fictitious patient who participates in a DMP. The patient is a 54-year-old woman with type 2 diabetes and COPD. She has a leg ulcer and moderate retinopathy. The patient is also moderately obese (BMI of 27). She has been unemployed for three years, receives social assistance benefits, and lives on her own.

Being unemployed, the patient would normally be covered under the statutory SHI scheme. She can therefore register voluntarily with her family physician to take part in the DMP programmes covering type 2 diabetes, asthma and COPD. This is conditional on suitable DMPs being offered in the region where the patient lives. If the patient's family physician does not participate in DMPs, but she wishes to join, she has the option of changing to another physician.

According to the regulations, treatment within the DMP begins with a thorough briefing on the programme, when the coordinating physician and the patient jointly set treatment goals for both her diabetes and COPD. Pharmaceuticals are prescribed according to the regulating framework which identifies the preferred substances for the treatment of type 2 diabetes and COPD. Any deviations from these procedures must be explained to the patient.

The family physician coordinates the patient's care. In this case, because of the patient's retinopathy, the family physician refers her to an ophthalmologist for an examination. The patient is also referred to a foot clinic for her leg ulcer and possible consequential damage to her legs and feet. She will be referred to a diabetes specialist when, for example, a target blood pressure value of below 140/90 mmHg or an individually agreed HbA1c value is not achieved, or when a change of treatment from oral anti-diabetic drugs to insulin becomes necessary. The patient is referred to a hospital (which should participate in the DMP) in the case of hypoglycaemia or diabetic ketoacidosis or if infection of her foot is suspected.

The asthma and COPD DMP stipulates referral to specialists when treatment results are unsatisfactory in spite of intensified therapy, when long-term treatment with oral steroids is required or when there are secondary disorders. Referral to a hospital is required in the case of a life-threatening exacerbation or significant deterioration of COPD in spite of initial treatment. After specialist treatment, the patient returns to the care of her family physician.

Monitoring is documented on a quarterly or half-yearly basis, at registration and at examination appointments, for both the diabetes and the asthma and COPD DMP. These data are recorded centrally and processed by the contract partners in the DMP, so as to optimize management of DMP patients in terms of regular follow-up and quality assurance.

The patient is required to participate actively in DMPs, for example in recommended education programmes; she will also receive two information brochures after initial registration, on diabetes and on asthma/COPD. Failure to participate in the programme can lead to cancellation of her registration with the DMP by her health insurance fund. However, active participation may be rewarded by additional benefits, such as exemption from the quarterly practice fee, or a reduction in the prescription fee for pharmaceuticals.

The DMP guidelines do not specifically refer to the particular social situation of the patient (in this case, unemployment). However, this is taken into consideration via the individual risk assessment required as part of the DMP and through the joint coordination of treatment goals. In addition, the coordinating physician always has the option of taking measures that apply in the usual care process.

Health system features supporting programmes

Targets, standards and guidelines

The regulatory framework for DMPs sets out standards and measures for quality assurance. Regional DMP agreements include requirements for the participation of family physicians in private practice, for providers of secondary health care services and for inpatient facilities.

Thus, participating family physicians are required to meet defined personal training standards (such as participation in further training on diabetes) and infrastructure requirements (such as availability of a training room). In addition, service providers are obliged to attend further training events and/or quality groups on a regular basis. Specialists have to acquire certain qualifications in order to qualify for participation in a DMP; for example, a specialist in a diabetes DMP must be formally recognized as a diabetologist in line with the requirements set out by the German Diabetes Society. Hospitals have to follow similar requirements.

Regional DMP contract partners verify whether physicians and specialists meet the requirements for participation and regular further training. However, the qualification standards for coordinating physicians are generally comparatively low. This is because it was considered important to not intimidate physicians with a nationwide roll-out of the programme by setting out excessively high demands for qualification and thus excluding too many physicians from potential participation.

Documentation of the course of treatment forms the basis for quality assurance by the contracting partners. The extent of the information to be documented is clearly defined and includes, alongside administrative data, information on the patient's condition and test results, current medication, patient education undertaken, and agreed treatment targets. This information is used to measure progress against DMP quality targets (Box 5.2), to generate feedback reports for individual practices and to issue reminders.

Against the background of quality targets as described in Box 5.2, DMPs must also set out measures to be taken if targets are not achieved. This is documented in feedback reports drawn up for every DMP physician. Service providers (that is, participating physicians and hospitals) that repeatedly contravene the programme's guidelines may receive a warning and may ultimately be excluded from further participation in the DMP. Achievement of quality targets is monitored at regional level by the DMP contract partners.

Several regional DMP partners have published quality reports which are also available through the World Wide Web (for example, AOK Baden-

> **Box 5.2 Quality targets in disease management programmes**
>
> In line with the regulatory framework, the contracting partners of a regional disease management programme (DMP) have to formulate quantifiable quality targets for the DMP in the following areas:
>
> - treatment requirements according to evidence-based guidelines (for example, the proportion of patients in the DMP diabetes with blood pressure under 140/90 mm Hg);
> - adherence to quality-assured and efficient pharmacological treatment (for example, the proportion of patients in the coronary heart disease DMP with myocardial infarction and those receiving treatment with beta-blockers);
> - cooperation between levels of care (for example, the number of patients in the DMP diabetes who are regularly referred for ophthalmological examinations);
> - adherence to the requirements for structural quality (for example, the proportion of participating physicians whose eligibility for participation is regularly checked);
> - completeness, availability and quality of documentation (for example, the proportion of patients who have been correctly registered with the DMP);
> - active participation of the patient (for example, the proportion of patients who take part in a recommended education programme).

Württemberg 2006, AOK Bayern 2005, AOK Rheinland-Pfalz 2005, Gemeinsame Einrichtung Thüringen 2005, Nordrheinische Gemeinsame Einrichtung Disease-Management-Programme GbR 2006). These reports usually contain the numbers of participating service providers and of patients registered with the DMPs in the respective region, as well as summarizing to what extent key quality targets have been achieved. The presentation of a quality report is a precondition for the reaccreditation of programmes through the Federal Insurance Office, which takes place three years after initial accreditation.

Health care workforce and capacity

DMPs in Germany operate within the existing system of statutory SHI and do not fundamentally alter the overall delivery structure that is characteristic of the German health care system; however, they have introduced minor medical and organizational changes designed to improve the care of patients with chronic disease(s).

One new element that differs from the usual care provided outside DMPs is that physicians and other organizations cannot automatically take part in DMPs. Instead, participating parties (physician(s) or hospital(s)) are required to submit a formal declaration that they meet the requirements outlined earlier. One other new element concerns the coordinating role of the family physician in the care of those with chronic disease(s), which has been strengthened through the introduction of DMPs. Thus, the boundaries to the secondary care level (specialists or hospitals) have been set out more clearly, including the tasks to be undertaken at each level. Again, these elements are not present in the usual system of care. Yet, at the same time, the qualifications required of service providers are still heavily orientated towards the physician-dominated structures that are characteristic of the German health care system. The setting in which chronic care takes place has also remained largely unchanged following the introduction of DMPs.

The involvement of nurses and nonmedical health professions has traditionally been low in the German health care system and this has not been changed by DMPs. DMPs thus continue to concentrate on physicians in their role as service providers, while other health professionals are not directly involved.

Financial management and incentives

In order to make structured health care programmes an attractive option for the health insurance funds, the DMPs were attached to the Risk Structure Compensation Scheme (RSA) (Box 5.1). The RSA was introduced in the mid-1990s as a means to reallocate revenue among statutory SHI funds so as to balance differences in risk profiles, and hence also expenditure on the population insured in a given fund.

The legal framework for DMPs stipulates that health insurance funds should receive an equalization payment for each insured person treated in a DMP, conditional upon the patient being registered with an accredited DMP. However, payments for each insured person to the RSA scheme have not been increased, which means that the equalization payments for non-registered patients were simultaneously reduced. As a consequence, health insurance funds with a large number of patients with chronic disease that succeed in registering most of them with a DMP will benefit from the equalization payments. Conversely, those funds that insure largely young and/or healthy patients or funds that fail to motivate a large number of their patients to register with a DMP will receive smaller transfer sums from the equalization scheme. Thus, by linking DMPs to the RSA scheme, health insurance funds have been provided with a substantial financial incentive to offer DMPs and to motivate their insurees to take part in these programmes. The additional costs incurred by health insurance funds to meet administration and documentation requirements as set out in the DMP regulations have been estimated at €85 per patient per year (Anonymous 2004).

At the same time, DMPs provide considerable financial incentives to service providers, as providers receive reimbursement for disease-specific education programmes for registered patients. They also receive additional compensation for the registration of an insured person into a DMP and for the regular production of standardized DMP documentation. On average, a coordinating physician receives an additional €75 per patient per year for the registration of the patient and for drawing up the necessary documentation (Anonymous 2004). Additional payments for participating physicians are usually limited to these flat rates and to fees for providing patient education programmes. All other medical services provided within DMPs are reimbursed as per the usual care system, through standard agreements independent of the DMPs.

As noted earlier, patients may also benefit from financial incentives when participating in DMPs; however, this is determined by the individual health insurance fund they are registered with. Incentives may include (partial) exemption from the quarterly practice fee of €10 or a reduced level of other co-payments, for example for pharmaceuticals.

Evaluation and lessons learned

DMPs in Germany were introduced to enhance the care of those with chronic disease(s) and to control the costs of care, by improving the quality of care through a structured course of treatment, providing patients with information and ensuring their active participation (Box 5.3).

In a relatively short period of time, Germany succeeded in introducing DMPs for breast cancer, type 2 diabetes and coronary heart disease throughout the country. This is mainly because DMPs were linked to the RSA, as outlined earlier, thereby providing financial incentives for health insurance funds and service providers. At the same time, this linkage also gave cause for concern. Thus, DMP documentation is not only used for quality assurance, but also as evidence to justify equalization payments between the health insurance funds. Payments are generated every time a patient is registered and every time DMP documentation is drawn up. Therefore, not only must the documentation meet medical criteria, but it must also withstand legal scrutiny. In practice, this has often led to a situation where formal programme requirements (resulting from the linkage to the RSA) have been difficult to implement in day-to-day health care provision. This has in effect led to a formalization of DMPs, with little scope for flexibility at local level. One concern has been that – because of the financial incentive linked to patients joining a DMP – health insurance funds may have focused unduly on recruiting insurees for registration in DMPs, rather than on the actual quality of care provided to high-risk patients.

> **Box 5.3 Formal evaluation criteria of disease management programmes in Germany**
>
> The regulatory framework has stipulated that disease management programmes (DMPs) are to be evaluated formally. The main goals of the statutory evaluation are to verify that the targets of the programme are reached, that the criteria for registration are adhered to and to assess the costs of care within DMPs (Bundesversicherungsamt 2007). The minimum requirements for the evaluation of the programmes were set out in the corresponding legislative and regulatory provisions, set out by the Federal Insurance Office in cooperation with the health insurance funds (Bundesversicherungsamt 2005). The costs of evaluation are borne by the health insurance funds.
>
> Evaluation requirements include a basic demographic characterization of participating patients and number of participating service providers. Taking diabetes as an example, the primary end-points of evaluations were defined as follows: death, heart attack, stroke, renal replacement therapy, amputation and blindness. The following were selected as secondary endpoints: diabetic nephropathy, neuropathy, diabetic foot disease, peripheral arterial disease and diabetic retinopathy. Further aspects are the patient's weight, smoking status, HbA1c levels, medication and participation in education programmes, along with patient-reported quality of life as assessed by questionnaires. Evaluations should also reflect on the costs of treatment in the various sectors, including administrative costs and the costs of quality assurance.
>
> The evaluation period is three years, during which three quality reports should be produced: after one year, 18 months and three years, and findings have recently been made available (AOK-Bundesverband 2007). However, in its current format, the statutory evaluation does not enable assessment of whether the newly introduced DMPs indeed make a difference to patient outcomes as compared to "usual" care. In 2005–2006, health insurance funds therefore commissioned additional scientific evaluations of two DMPs (diabetes and coronary heart disease). Initial findings of the type 2 diabetes DMP evaluation seem to indicate improved quality of chronic illness care as reported by enrolled patients, compared to those receiving usual care, although a relatively modest response rate and the cross-sectional nature of the evaluation restricts generalization of the findings (Szecsenyi et al. 2008). An observational study of patients enrolled in a coronary heart disease DMP also indicates improved patient-reported quality of care compared to usual care, although actual health outcomes were not found to differ significantly (Gapp et al. 2008).

The GBA has examined the effectiveness of the individual medical components of the DMPs. However, there was little attempt to study systematically the combination of various components and their application in practice, in particular as it relates to data flow (documentation, registration, validity checks, data analysis) before nationwide roll-out of the entire programme. Thus, there was little discussion about whether the individual measures would be acceptable to patients and service providers and whether there was a suitable organizational and financial framework in place for the implementation of these measures. Not surprisingly, perhaps, there were considerable initial difficulties in the implementation of the DMPs, particularly with respect to documentation, along with data registration and use.

From the provider perspective, there was particular concern in relation to the extent of paperwork required for patient administration. In particular, the regular DMP documentation, data recording and subsequent validation have proved difficult to translate into daily practice. Also, forms which had not been tested in practice, inconsistent and partly flawed guidelines, and regulations on deadlines not compatible with health care practice have led to a heavy workload for service providers. It is important to note that the external evaluation of DMPs commissioned by the health insurance funds, (Box 5.3), will not examine the extent to which medical and organizational guidelines set out in the regulatory framework can actually be implemented in day-to-day practice, or indeed whether they can be implemented at all.

At the same time, the proposed quality assurance measures, such as the production of feedback reports for physicians, have not been carried out to the same extent in all regions. Service providers may thus be under the impression that the disproportionate workload required for documentation is not justified by a corresponding benefit for either individual patients or the service providers themselves.

Another requirement which has been found difficult to implement in practice is the active participation of patients, a central objective of DMPs. In line with regulatory requirements, lack of active participation on the part of the patient can be assumed when, within a period of three years, two successive sets of documentation are not received. Yet, in practice it is not uncommon for documentation to be missing for variety of reasons which are not always related to a lack of willingness to participate on the part of the patient. Consequently, the registration of large numbers of patients would have to be rescinded, even though in reality they were actually engaged with DMP activities.

There is also concern, mostly among providers, that programmes could impede clinical freedom in decision-making and thus lead to poor-quality health care. Service providers have also heavily criticized the fact that some medical data on individual patients have been made available to health insurance funds, a procedure that has hitherto not been customary in the German health care system. It was argued that making these data available to the health insurance funds would threaten the trust between the physician and the patient.

As noted earlier, the principles of medical care in DMPs were developed by the GBA, where representatives of service providers and of purchasers (that is, health insurance funds) have an equal number of votes. Nonmedical stakeholders are thus deciding on medical content for the first time. Simultaneously, medical policy is being issued in the form of a regulation, and is thus for the first time the subject of normative rulings by the State. In this way, the introduction of DMPs has led to the legislature playing a direct and detailed role in determining health service provision in Germany. Service providers in particular are concerned that the DMPs could lead to a de-professionalization of physicians and mark the initiation of a state-controlled health care system.

The process of external evaluation of DMPs has also been the subject of controversy. The fact that no study has been carried out to compare the care provided in DMPs with usual care is a matter of particular criticism: the chosen form of evaluation makes it impossible to judge whether the newly introduced programmes will indeed make a difference to patient outcomes as compared to usual care. In addition, in their current form, the German DMPs target individual chronic disease only and do not address the problem of multi-morbidity, which means that these DMPs are open to the criticism that they favour individual diseases in a relatively arbitrary way.

Investing in the future

DMPs in Germany have at their disposal various measures to improve the care of patients with chronic disease. These include the definition of medical processes; requirements for the participation of service providers; mandatory further training; the active participation of patients; structured documentation; quality assurance instruments, such as feedback reports and external scientific evaluation; as well as an adapted financing system. In this way, the DMPs offer an opportunity for the best available evidence to be integrated into day-to-day health care in Germany.

However, there is a persuasive argument that nationwide introduction of DMPs should have been preceded by a pilot scheme to ascertain the extent to which programmes are able to contribute to better care for patients, and whether the structural components of the programmes can be implemented in routine practice.

An effective restructuring of care for those with chronic conditions needs to go beyond stipulations made by the regulatory framework, as is the case at the time of writing. Successful implementation of such a programme requires engagement with the actual providers of care, backed by political and institutional support at local level by purchasers (that is, representatives of the health insurance funds), the KVs, medical associations and the regional opinion leaders among physicians. Implementation is unlikely to achieve its full potential if health insurance funds are predominately interested in optimizing their revenue, and medical associations merely insist on maintaining physicians' privileges.

The German DMPs, as presently structured, have not required any fundamental alteration to existing structures in the German health care system. Services continue to be provided within the existing delivery structure, comprising family physicians, specialists in private practice, and hospitals. The integration of nonmedical health professionals into the care system, which has led to considerable improvements in chronic care elsewhere, is not being promoted within the current DMP system. Similarly, the continued sectoral barriers between inpatient and ambulatory care, caused in part by the differing financing structures, are unlikely to be overcome by DMPs. Thus, one of the greatest challenges for the German health care system will remain the development of a multidisciplinary reorganization of the care of patients with chronic disease, oriented towards a generic model.

Yet, despite these challenges, there remains a clear consensus that DMPs are an important tool for improving the care of those with chronic disease(s). Simplification of requirements for DMP documentation and data flows should contribute to reducing the administrative burden that hampers DMPs at the time of writing. To better address multi-morbidity within the existing structure of DMPs, the legislature has now mandated the GBA to develop modules for obesity and cardiac failure that would supplement the existing DMPs. An obese patient with coronary heart disease who also suffers from heart failure could then be treated in the coronary heart disease DMP with supplementary modules on cardiac failure and obesity.

The financial incentives for improvement of chronic care will also change in the coming years. Work is being carried out at the time of writing to reform the RSA outlined earlier, expected to take effect from 1 January 2009. This will take account of the actual health status of the insured population covered by a health insurance fund and would thus be directly taken into account in the RSA for the calculation of the equalization payments between different funds. In contrast, the participation of patients in DMPs will no longer be taken into consideration in the RSA from 2009 onwards. However, because policy-makers will continue to promote the expansion and further development of DMPs, health insurance funds will receive a uniform flat rate (€180) for every DMP patient. Strengths and weaknesses of the key components of chronic disease management in Germany are presented in Table 5.2.

Table 5.2 *Chronic disease management in Germany: strengths and weaknesses*

	Strengths	Weaknesses	Opportunities	Threats
Consistency of policies	DMPs are consistent with current models for chronic disease management including focus on self-care and evidence-based recommendations, quality assurance and evaluation	DMPs place considerable administrative burden on providers The DMP accreditation system imposes a high administrative burden on central authorities The system in place does not allow flexibility to adapt DMPs to regional health needs Focus on individual diseases: DMPs do not take sufficient account of the health care needs of patients with multiple conditions	DMPs contribute to structured care for people with chronic conditions Greatly enhanced use of evidence in chronic disease management Increased emphasis on self-management / patient education Opportunities to greatly advance quality assurance system in the health care sector	DMPs were rolled out across Germany without prior testing in a controlled pilot DMPs do not address some of the fundamental weaknesses of the general framework of the German statutory system (e.g. training; separation of ambulatory and hospital sector) DMPs mainly involve the medical profession, there is no systematic development of nonmedical roles
Influence of electoral cycles	DMPs are generally supported by all political parties	Financial incentives provided by risk equalization scheme are not unanimously supported by the political stakeholders Potential influence of political stakeholders on clinical contents of DMPs	Current efforts among key stakeholders to simplify the administrative processes within DMPs Increased efforts to shift focus to health care needs of people with multiple conditions	(Potential) amendments to the financing structure of DMPs (i.e. disengaging from the risk equalization scheme) is likely to threaten the sustainability of DMPs

(cont.)

Table 5.2 *(cont.)*

	Strengths	Weaknesses	Opportunities	Threats
Impact of institutional framework	Responsibilities in and requirements for DMPs are clearly defined Accreditation of DMPs is in place Countrywide introduction of DMPs supported by the insurance funds as a key stakeholder	There is some resistance to DMPs by physicians' associations	Rapid and countrywide introduction of DMPs DMPs are regularly reviewed and updated	Lack of uniform support from key stakeholders or vested interests of individual stakeholders
Impact of macroeconomic conditions/ constraints	Current link between DMP financing and risk equalization schemes provides financial incentives for insurance funds to promote the introduction of DMPs	There is some debate whether enhanced activity of insurance funds in promoting DMPs is because of the financial incentives linked to their implementation rather than a genuine interest in improving the quality of care Linking DMPs to the risk equalization scheme has greatly increased the administrative burden	Linking DMPs to the risk equalization scheme has greatly supported their extensive implementation across Germany	Amendments to the financing structure of DMPs (i.e. disengaging from the risk equalization scheme) is likely to threaten the sustainability of DMPs
Influence of other agencies / policies	Policies are well informed by international trends	Implementation of international models without sufficient evaluation of appropriateness/ transferability to the German context	System of external evaluation of DMPs in place	Potential regional variation in terms of population need Insufficient consideration of regional requirements

Source: Authors' own compilation.
Note: DMP: Disease management programme.

References

Anonymous (2004). Disease Management kostet 160 Euro pro Patient [Disease management costs 160 euros per patient] *Ärzte Zeitung*, 20 September 2004.

AOK-Bundesverband (2007). *Zukunftsmodell DMP. Erfolge und Perspektiven der Programme fuer chronisch Kranke*. Berlin, AOK-Bundesverband.

AOK Baden-Württemberg (2006). *Qualitätsbericht Disease-Management-Programm Diabetes mellitus Typ 2: Berichtszeitraum 01.10.2003 – 31.12.2005*. Stuttgart, AOK Baden-Württemberg.

AOK Bayern (2005). *DMP-Qualitätsbericht für die Diagnose Diabetes mellitus Typ 2: Zeitraum: 01.01.2004 – 30.06.2005*. Munchen, AOK Bayern.

AOK Rheinland-Pfalz (2005). *Qualitätsbericht 2005: Das strukturierte Behandlungsprogramm „Diabetes mellitus Typ 2" der AOK – Die Gesundheitskasse in Rheinland-Pfalz*. Eisenberg, AOK Rheinland-Pfalz (http://www.aok-dmp.de/PDF/Qualitaetssicherungsbericht%20Diabetes%20mellitus%20Typ%202%20-%202005.pdf, accessed 19 December 2006).

Bundesministerium der Justiz (2008). Verordnung über das Verfahren zum Risikostrukturausgleich in der gesetzlichen Krankenversicherung (Risikostruktur-Ausgleichsverordnung – RSAV) [web site]. Berlin, Bundesministerium der Justiz (http://www.bundesrecht.juris.de/rsav/BJNR005500994.html, accessed May 2008).

Bundesministerium für Gesundheit (2006a). Strukturierte Behandlungsprogramme [web site]. Berlin, Bundesministerium für Gesundheit (http://www.die-gesundheitsreform.de/glossar/strukturierte_behandlungsprogramme.html, accessed 19 December 2006).

Bundesministerium für Gesundheit (2006b) [web site]. Gesetzliche Krankenkassen in Deutschland 2006. Berlin, Bundesministerium für Gesundheit (http://www.die-gesundheitsreform.de/presse/infografiken/pdf/infografik_gkv_brd_2006.pdf, accessed 19 December 2006).

Bundesministerium für Gesundheit (2006c) [web site]. Mehr als zwei Millionen Menschen profitieren von strukturierten Behandlungsprogrammen für chronisch Kranke. Berlin, Bundesministerium für Gesundheit (http://www.die-gesundheitsreform.de/presse/pressemitteilung/dokumente/2006_1/pm_2006-02-01-012.html, accessed 19 December 2006).

Bundesversicherungsamt (2005) [web site]. Leitfaden für die Antragstellung zur Zulassung strukturierter Behandlungsprogramme. Bonn, Bundesversicherungsamt (http://www.bva.de/Fachinformationen/Dmp/leitfaden.pdf, accessed 19 December 2006).

Bundesversicherungsamt (2007). *Kriterien des Bundesversicherungsamtes zur Evaluation strukturierter Behandlungsprogramme.* Bonn, Bundesversicherungsamt (http://www.bundesversicherungsamt.de/nn_1046154/DE/DMP/Downloads/Downloads__Evaluation__gesamt,templateId=raw,property=publicationFile.pdf/Downloads_Evaluation_gesamt.pdf, accessed May 2008).

Bundesversicherungsamt (2008) [web site]. Zulassung der Disease Management Programme (DMP) durch das Bundesversicherungsamt (BVA). Bonn, Bundesversicherungsamt (http://www.bundesversicherungsamt.de/nn_1046154/DE/DMP/dmp__node.html?__nnn=true#doc1046158bodyText7, accessed May 2008).

Busse R, Riesberg A (2004). Health care systems in transition: Germany. *Health Systems in Transition*, 6(9):1–234.

Ettelt S et al. (2006). *Health care outside hospital. Accessing generalist and specialist care in eight countries.* Copenhagen, WHO Regional Office for Europe.

Gapp O et al. (2008). Disease management programmes for patients with coronary heart disease. An empirical study of German programmes. *Health Policy*, in press.

Gawlik C (2005). Aufgabe und Rolle des Bundesversicherungsamtes (BVA). In: Tophoven C, Sell S (eds). *Disease-Management-Programme. Die Chance nutzen.* Köln, Deutscher Ärzte-Verlag:31–40.

Gemeinsame Einrichtung Thüringen (2005). *Qualitätsbericht. Disease-Management-Programm Diabetes mellitus Typ 2.* Weimar, Gemeinsame Einrichtung Thüringen.

Hilfer S, Riesberg A, Egger B (2007). *Adapting social security health care systems to trends in chronic disease: Germany.* Geneva, International Social Secirity Assocation (ISSA) Technical Commission on Medical Care and Sickness Insurance.

Kaiser T, Jennen E, Sawicki PT (2003). *Entscheidungsgrundlage zur evidenzbasierten Diagnostik und Therapie bei Disease Management Programmen für Koronare Herzkrankheit, stabile Angina pectoris.* Köln, DIeM – Institut für evidenzbasierte Medizin.

Kaiser T, Krones R, Sawicki PT (2003a). *Entscheidungsgrundlage zur evidenzbasierten Diagnostik und Therapie bei Disease Management Programmen für Diabetes mellitus Typ 2.* Köln, DIeM – Instiut für evidenzbasierte Medizin.

Kaiser T, Krones R, Sawicki PT (2003b). *Entscheidungsgrundlage zur evidenzbasierten Diagnostik und Therapie bei Disease Management Programmen für Diabetes mellitus Typ 1.* Köln, DIeM – Institut für evidenzbasierte Medizin.

Lauterback KW et al. (2001). *Disease Management in Deutschland: Voraussetzungen, Rahmenbedingungen, Faktoren zur Entwicklung, Implementierung und Evaluation.* Köln, Institut für Gesundheitsökonomie und Klinische Epidemiologie der Universität zu Köln (http://www.uk-koeln.de/kai/igmg/guta/GutachtenDMP.pdf, accessed 19 December 2006).

Nordrheinische Gemeinsame Einrichtung Disease-Management-Programme GbR (2006). *Qualitätssicherungsbericht 2005 Disease-Management-Programme in Nordrhein.* Düsseldorf, Nordrheinische Gemeinsame Einrichtung Disease-Management-Programme GbR.

Sell S (2005). Disease-Management-Programme – von der Idee zum Gesetz [Disease management programme. In: Tophoven C, Sell S (eds). *Disease-Management-Programme. Die Chance nutzen.* Köln, Deutscher Ärzte-Verlag:1–18.

Szecsenyi J et al. (2008). German diabetes disease management programmes are appropriate for restructuring care according to the chronic care model: an evaluation with the patient assessment of chronic illness care instrument. *Diabetes Care,* 31:1150–1154.

Chapter 6
The Netherlands

Eveline Klein Lankhorst, Cor Spreeuwenberg

Context

The Dutch health care system builds on a long tradition in which charities were responsible for caring for the sick and disabled. The principal system of mandatory health insurance was introduced during German occupation of the country in the Second World War. This system, subsequently defined by the 1964 Sickness Fund Act, provided coverage for all those below a certain income level. It was replaced in the reform of 2006 by the Health Insurance Act, which made health insurance compulsory for all residents. The new Act aimed to ensure access to essential curative health care for all residents, improve the quality of health care and reduce health care expenditure by strengthening market mechanisms in the health care system and by promoting competition.

Under the new system, all residents are entitled to the same comprehensive package of essential curative health services, which they purchase from private health insurers, replacing the previous non-profit-making (public) sickness funds. The system is financed through (1) a nominal premium to be paid by the insured person to the individual insurance fund and which may vary between different funds; and (2) additional income-related premiums collected from all citizens above 18 years, redistributed to the individual health insurers along with a "risk equalization scheme" to compensate for differences in the risk profiles of the insured population. Employers are obliged to compensate their employees partly for their income-related premiums. Where the nominal premium is excessive relative to income, individuals are entitled to a rebate from the tax authorities, which collect income-related contributions (Ministry of Health Welfare and Sport 2006, Maarse 2006).

Health insurers are required to accept every resident but the insured may change funds if they so wish. This is thought to create incentives for insurers to provide the best package possible under the conditions of a quasi-market. Insured individuals may choose between receiving benefits in kind or reimbursement of expenses. From January 2008, the no-claims bonus system has been replaced by a compulsory own contribution system, collected by the health insurer, of up to €150 for each insured person over the age of 18 years. Those with a chronic condition receive a rebate of €47.

The Government determines coverage and entitlements to essential services within the framework of the Health Insurance Act, according to the principles of accessibility, affordability and quality. Additional supplementary insurance can be purchased for services not covered by the package of essential services. Insurance premiums are determined by the insurers, with payments negotiated between insurers and health care providers.

An essential characteristic of the reformed system is that, because of the central role of private health insurance, it is based on private law but incorporates strong elements of public law. This is vital for safeguarding the social character of the Dutch health insurance scheme (Ministry of Health Welfare and Sport 2006, Maarse 2006).

Health services are generally delivered by private providers in both the ambulatory and hospital sectors. Hospitals are traditionally owned and operated by private non-profit-making organizations.

The 2006 health reform also involved changing the previous relevant Exceptional Medical Expenses Act (AWBZ), which provided universal coverage for long-term care, including home care, nursing homes, mental health care, facilities for disabled people, and other preventive activities. Entitlements under the AWBZ to home care and social assistance, for example, are now covered by the Social Support Act (WMO), which supports municipalities in providing people with the means to remain as independent as possible. The premium is income dependent and collected as payroll tax.

As elsewhere, the rise in the number of people with chronic disease(s) presents a challenge to the financing and delivery of high-quality health care in the Netherlands. At present, the Dutch health system does not fully meet the requirements of those with chronic disease(s). While ensuring good access to health services, there remain numerous challenges in areas of prevention, continuity of care, cooperation and patient orientation.

Analysing the response

Approaches to chronic disease management

The concept of "transmural care" was introduced in 1994 in an attempt to overcome persistent barriers between ambulatory and acute services (Linden 2000, Vrijhoef 2002). The term "transmural" is derived from "intramural" care, or care inside a hospital or nursing home, and "extramural" care, which refers to primary care in general practice or home-based settings. Transmural care aims to link primary and secondary care; it has been defined as care geared towards the needs of the patient, provided on the basis of cooperation and coordination between general and specialized caregivers, with shared responsibilities and specification of delegated responsibilities (Vrijhoef 2002). Transmural care has been likened to shared care concepts in the United Kingdom and integrated care in the United States (Kodner & Spreeuwenberg 2002, Vrijhoef et al. 2001). The key objective was to improve quality of care by better coordinating primary and specialist care, and to enhance effectiveness, patient orientation, continuity, service availability and efficiency of care for the entire population.

Transmural care concepts in the Netherlands vary widely, with early approaches focusing on structural elements. Examples include enhancing cooperation between hospitals and GPs and the development of medical guidelines. Specialized nurses later became involved, broadening the scope of care by linking medical treatment with prevention, information, education, and social and psychological support. They also acted as transfer (or liaison) nurses, responsible for the preparation and planning of patient discharge, as well as advising and, in some cases, even supervising GPs, or transferring patients back into primary care after hospital treatment.

More recently, rehabilitation wards were created for patients who required temporary care after hospitalization. Also, advances in technology made it possible to transfer certain services that were previously restricted to the hospital setting into the patient's home. Over time, transmural care approaches became increasingly complex, as exemplified by the development of disease management programmes (such as the Matador programme as described in the following subsection), involving cooperation between a greater range of health care facilities and health professionals (Linden van der 2000, Spreeuwenberg et al. 2000).

The Matador programme

One example of a complex programme that has evolved from the transmural care projects of the 1990s is the Matador programme, the Maastricht

Fig. 6.1 *Care levels in the Matador programme*

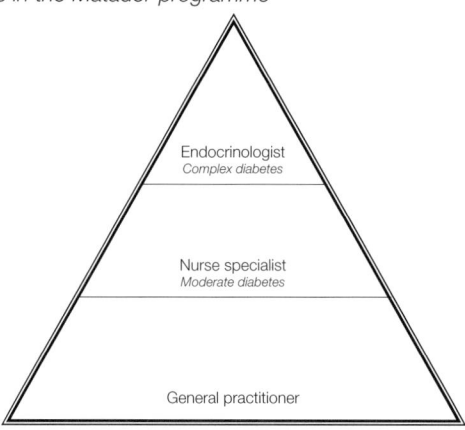

```
          /\
         /  \
        /Endo-\
       /crinologist\
      / Complex diabetes \
     /────────────\
    /              \
   /  Nurse specialist  \
  /   Moderate diabetes   \
 /──────────────\
/                        \
/   General practitioner   \
──────────────────
```

Source: Adapted from Maastricht Transmural Diabetes Organisation 2000.

Transmural Diabetes Organization. Its origins date back to 1981 when the Academic Hospital Maastricht (AZM) initiated a programme to enhance the diagnostic skills of GPs attached to the hospital. The programme was subsequently expanded to incorporate the development of common protocols and joint consultations involving specialists and GPs. In 1996 it began piloting a scheme to delegate tasks to nurses in primary care (that is, general practice) who had specialized in diabetes, asthma and COPD in an attempt to reduce the number of patients seen by medical specialists in outpatient settings. Following a successful evaluation, the programme was subsequently transformed into a disease management programme in which nurses have the primary responsibility for the treatment of patients with diabetes, asthma and/or COPD.

The Matador programme (subsequently the Maastricht Diabetes Care Group, see Box 6.1) was formally launched in January 2000 and is open to all GPs in the Maastricht region (Eijkelberg et al. 2001). It involves two main transfers of roles, from doctors to nurses and from hospital to primary care. In Maastricht, some services are provided in a newly established diabetes clinic which serves as the organizational and coordination centre of the Matador programme (Vrijhoef et al. 2001, Vrijhoef 2002).

All patients participating in the programme are registered with a GP. Each is supported by a core team comprising a GP, an endocrinologist and a specialist diabetes nurse. The core team is organized around the GP. Patients are stratified according to the severity of their condition and, based on defined criteria, those with complex cases are allocated to the endocrinologist, patients with unstable disease to the specialist nurse and the remainder to the GP (Fig. 6.1). The roles of the core team members are clearly defined and each team member has explicit responsibility for the patients allocated to them.

The endocrinologist supervises the specialist nurse and acts as a consultant to the GP and the specialist nurse; s/he also contributes to their specialized education. The nurse specialists supervise and act as a consultant to the GP in relation to diabetes care. In turn, the GP informs the nurse on other aspects related to the patient and of relevance to the care process. Members of the core team meet on a regular basis to discuss each patient's needs, although meetings involving all core teams are rare because of organizational difficulties. Core teams cooperate with other caregivers, such as dieticians, community nurses, podiatrists and ophthalmologists (Vrijhoef et al. 2001). At the time of writing approximately 60 GPs in the Maastricht region participated in the programme. There are comparable programmes for patients with COPD and asthma.

Patient treatment is based on a protocol, which comprises specific guidelines on diabetes care. Patients have quarterly consultations with a nurse specialist and every other year patients will also see an endocrinologist. This is very different from the situation in the past, when patients with diabetes would see an endocrinologist on a quarterly basis (Vrijhoef et al. 2001).

The specialist diabetes nurse also fulfils an active role in patient education (Maastricht Transmural Diabetes Organisation 2000, ZonMw 2006a). This has led to the creation of the Diabetes Interactive Education Programme (DIEP), designed to promote patient education and to assist those with diabetes to manage their own condition (DIEP 2008). The design of the programme was based in part on the observation that knowledge and ability to self-manage improve substantially when patients are seen by a specialist nurse (Pepels, Linden van der & Huijsman 2004, Vrijhoef 2002).

Distribution, uptake and coverage

It has been estimated that, since the introduction of the concept in the early 1990s, each hospital in the Netherlands has been involved in some form of transmural care, with 504 schemes being developed between 1996 and 2000 (Linden van der, Spreeuwenberg & Schrijvers 2001). Each transmural scheme involves an average of three health care organizations; these were mainly hospitals (involved in 98% of transmural care projects), home care organizations (75%), GPs (21%), nursing homes (22%), health insurance funds (18%) and patient organizations (12%), as well as health care professionals such as medical specialists (75%), hospital-based nurses (73%) and home care nurses (69%) (Linden van der, Spreeuwenberg & Schrijvers 2001). During the same period, approximately 10% of GPs in the Netherlands were involved in some form of disease management (Steuten et al. 2002). There is, however, little information about population coverage by transmural care schemes or other disease management initiatives.

As described earlier, in the Dutch health system each resident is entitled to essential health care, including access to services for chronic diseases. Thus, under the new Health Insurance Act, health insurance funds are not permitted to select their insured population but have to accept every resident in their area of activity. Insurers do, however, have some scope to introduce barriers by awarding premium reductions to people covered by an employer's collective contract and by introducing selection criteria for additional insurance, thereby indirectly selecting patients. In addition, while transmural care projects and coordinated approaches to disease management have been implemented across the country, some have been more successful and sustainable than others, potentially introducing inequalities, as successful programmes are limited to certain providers or regions.

A patient journey: the Netherlands

Here we describe a typical patient journey for a fictitious patient, a 54-year-old woman with type 2 diabetes and asthma. The patient is also moderately obese (BMI of 27), she has been unemployed for three years, receives social assistance benefits, and lives on her own.

In this example, the patient has received long-term asthma treatment with corticosteroids and she now reports to her respiratory specialist physician with visual disturbances and an ulcer on her left leg which will not heal. It is likely that the pulmonologist will carry out tests and diagnose her diabetes; s/he might also refer the patient directly to an internist or back to the GP. Diabetes is typically diagnosed opportunistically, as part of a routine consultation or when the patient visits a physician because of (an)other complaint(s). Only a few GPs systematically control the glucose-levels of patients considered at risk of diabetes.

Once the diabetes has been confirmed, the patient is likely to be initially treated by her GP, who will refer her to an ophthalmologist. The management of the leg ulcer depends on its localization and severity. The GP may refer her to the district nurse for dressing the ulcer. She may also be referred to a podiatrist or dermatologist. In the event that the respiratory specialist physician who saw the patient for her asthma referred her to an internist, she will receive treatment and will then be referred to a specialized nurse, a dietician, an ophthalmologist and a dermatologist.

The Dutch College of General Practitioners (NHG) guidelines propose a quarterly follow-up to measure HbA1c, urine, weight and blood pressure. The patient will also have thorough check-ups on an annual basis. The GP will allocate responsibility for her management to either her/himself, the practice nurse or a diabetes nurse specialist. As the patient also has asthma, it is likely that the GP may take on management of the patient. However, because of her specific social situation, the follow-up might be carried out by a nurse. The nurse also plays an important role in education and information, that is, by sharing information from the Dutch Diabetes Association, interactive programmes, brochures and leaflets as well as accessible support systems. Ideally the patient will be involved in the decision-making process.

In case of a complication, the patient is expected to call upon her GP. Normally the patient will be seen the same day. In serious cases the emergency services will be called upon. There is some experimentation with call centres and support systems to assess complications and so direct patients to the services they require.

Health system features supporting programmes

Targets, standards and guidelines

Rights and duties of health care professionals are set out in the Law on Professionals in Health Care (BiG), on Medical Treatment by Professionals (WGBO) and on the Prescription of Medicines (WGV). Other mechanisms are the accreditation of guidelines, standards, protocols and other professional norms.

Within the Matador programme described earlier, nurses performed duties that were formally outside their legally defined range of competencies. For instance, a nurse may change the dosage regime, but may not actually prescribe pharmaceuticals or refer patients to other health professionals. To overcome this barrier, new protocols extending the role(s) of nurses were submitted to the Dutch Health Care Inspectorate (IGZ), responsible for health care quality and health protection, to obtain written permission to carry out this experiment. While approaches of this kind are often used to overcome existing barriers between practice and law, they do raise concerns related to accountability and compliance with the law.

It is important to note, however, that delegating tasks to nurses that are formally outside their range of competencies is common practice. Some GPs will allow a nurse to refer patients on her/his own initiative, while others are far stricter in their interpretation of professional roles. This variation inevitably creates uncertainty among specialized nurses as to their role, leading to demands for a uniform framework that clarifies tasks and responsibilities for all parties involved.

The Dutch Institute for Health Care Improvement (CBO) develops instruments and methods for quality improvement and innovation, for example, evidence-based guidelines on chronic conditions, such as diabetes and COPD (Dutch Institute for Healthcare Improvement 2008). An example of such a guideline is the "guideline for COPD chain of care", which contains material to support the practice of health care providers engaged in the care of patients with COPD. Several organizations have contributed to the document, including the country's asthma charities, the Dutch Society of Doctors for Lung Diseases and Tuberculosis (NVALT), the NHG Asthma and COPD GPs consulting group (NHG-CAHAG) and the CBO. Guidelines addressing specific diseases are developed by the relevant organizations, depending on their expertise. A more recent development has been the development of care standards which combine the contents of care with care processes and organization. For example, the newly developed standards for COPD and vascular risk management use the Chronic Care Model (CCM) to describe the elements of care required for a specific health problem.

Health care workforce and capacity

One concern in the Dutch health care system has been its fragmented nature and decentralized governance, resulting in poor coordination of initiatives to support health care workers dealing with the care of patients with chronic disease (Mur-Veeman, Eijkelberg & Spreeuwenberg 2001). In the 1990s the National Commission for the Chronically Ill (NCCZ) made the case for new intermediary roles for nurses (between medicine and nursing) in the field of chronic care. Several health care organizations have responded by developing in-service training programmes for nurses to take on some roles traditionally carried out by physicians. There were initially no formal educational programmes and various titles were used, such as nurse specialist, specialist diabetes nurse, advanced clinical nurse, nurse practitioner or physician assistant, although these titles have so far not been recognized formally. In 2004 the Minister of Health appointed a steering committee (MOBG) to consider the modernization of professional training in health care, with the aim of defining roles, competencies and qualifications.

While special education programmes for nurses have been developed and implemented, the training of physicians, medical specialists and GPs has remained focused on direct curative services at the expense of the organization of care, health promotion and health education, in particular with reference to chronic disease. Maastricht University has developed a multidisciplinary Master's-level course to train an "advanced clinical nurse specialist", a degree which has so far not been available at university level in the Netherlands.

Although recognized by the Accreditation Organisation of the Netherlands and Flanders (*Nederlands-Vlaamse Accreditatieorganisatie*, NVAO), the Master's programme has met with resistance from professional organizations and schools for higher education and has not been implemented.

In summary, the lack of a clear framework has prevented the development of formal education programmes related specifically to chronic care (Vrijhoef 2002). Development has also been hampered by a tradition of competition between professional schools of nursing and universities that train physicians, along with continued resistance from professional organizations. Thus, nursing organizations were concerned that nurses would be given responsibility for additional medical tasks without appropriate corresponding remuneration and without having an independent and legally regulated status.

The development of transmural care in the early 1990s has impacted on the health care workforce in the Netherlands through the expansion of the roles of nurses, as indicated earlier, but also through the introduction of teamwork among health professionals. Thus, GPs were no longer exclusively responsible for all tasks in a primary care setting, but rather shared tasks such as management, organization, infrastructure, professional development, direct patient care and education with other professionals. While GPs remain responsible for diagnosis, early treatment, co-morbidity and complications, in many cases nurses have taken on primary responsibility for people with minor illnesses and those with chronic disease. This implies a shift between the professions working in primary care, with more nurses and fewer physicians.

The aforementioned MOBG is tasked with modernizing professional structures and medical training. Although professional groups seek to protect their position by influencing the MOBG's decisions, the reality is that the demand for all health care professionals will increase.

One other instrument influencing the composition of the workforce is the admission to medical training through a "numerus fixus": the Ministry of Education determines the number of new medical students to be admitted to university each year, based on the current number of practising physicians and policy considerations. The Government may also limit admission to specialties such as general practice and internal medicine.

The call for a shift in responsibility for chronic care from physicians to nurses originates from the evidence that the care provided by nurses for patients with chronic disease is of at least similar quality to that provided by physicians and may be more cost-effective. However, while medical schools have little difficulty attracting students, professional nursing schools do. Yet, the primary care sector offers a broad spectrum of challenging new roles for the nursing profession and nursing schools provide a range of graduate programmes. That said, these programmes are only likely to attract sufficient student numbers if professional status and working conditions associated with the new roles are also enhanced. One response has been to upgrade nursing tasks and to ensure that less-qualified personnel cover basic nursing tasks.

Financial management and incentives

New approaches in the field of chronic care are being financed for the most part by health insurers. The 2006 Health Insurance Act has facilitated new contracting methods between providers and health insurance funds. For example, GPs may form diabetes care groups that commit to providing care for patients with diabetes, based on the principles of disease management, as per the system in place in the Maastricht region (Box 6.1). The diabetes care group acts as the contractor with a health insurance fund and sub-contracts GPs, medical specialists, diabetes nurses and others. Payment is carried out per item of service directly or indirectly provided by the programme. These new payment arrangements encourage GPs to keep patients out of hospital by treating them within the community. At the same time, however, these new arrangements potentially discourage cooperation between primary and secondary care levels.

Insurers can potentially influence future developments of programmes for specific groups of people with chronic disease and, in some regions, they have

> **Box 6.1 Financing arrangements for diabetes care in the Matador programme**
>
> Before the introduction of the 2006 health care reform in the Netherlands, the Matador programme was financed from different sources. General practitioners (GPs), endocrinologists, other medical specialists, dieticians and other health professionals were paid in accordance with the previous system (per person or salary), while for specialist diabetes nurses a special arrangement had to be put in place. Formally employed by the hospital, they were "seconded" to a home care organization. Since the nurses provided care in the community, it was permissible for the home care organizations to claim reimbursement for these services under the previous Exceptional Medical Expenses Act (AWBZ).
>
> Following the reform of the health insurance system, the Matador programme was transformed into a diabetes care group in which all regional GPs participate. To reduce costs and to reduce specialization within general practice, patients with diabetes are now treated by nurse practitioners, who have received general training in the care of chronic patients. Specialist diabetes nurses are responsible for patients with more complex conditions and act as consultants to nurse practitioners. The Matador programme is still housed within the Academic Hospital Maastricht (AZM), and its cooperation with the departments of endocrinology and the scientific evaluators has been maintained.

played a pivotal role in programme design. In the future they will also look to develop cost-effective programmes.

Insurers are currently considering encouraging patients to participate in the chronic care programmes by reducing the insurance premium to be paid by participants. The Government has asked ZonMw, a national institute responsible for evaluation and implementation of health care innovations, to encourage the development of new programmes by providing financial incentives to 10 "front runners", while ZonMw will undertake scientific evaluation of the selected programmes. It also provides practical support by subsidizing and evaluating certain chronic disease programmes, such as the Matador programme.

Evaluation and lessons learned

In the 1990s many hospitals took initiatives in the field of "transmural" care. Criteria for judging the success of these initiatives have included a clear vision, ambition, the setting of achievable goals and the capacity to bridge differences across sectors and among professions. The Government strengthened activities in transmural care by establishing the NCCZ (now the National Panel for Chronically Ill People and Handicapped Persons (*Nationaal panel Chronisch zieken en Gehandicapten* (NPCG), established in 1997)) (NPCG 2008), identifying financial support and carrying out scientific evaluations.

As described earlier, transmural care projects varied widely in the type of approach chosen and the range of professionals and institutions involved. It was also expected that projects would be transformed into sustainable and robust programmes with a sound financial base, thus requiring project leaders to identify appropriate financing mechanisms to ensure sustainability. As a consequence, the effectiveness of projects has varied widely. Successful initiatives were often limited to innovative groups in regions with academic centres or large hospitals that were able to combine meaningful innovations with scientific evaluations.

Some transmural care projects have been transformed in formal disease management programmes. However, disease management is still a relatively new phenomenon in the Netherlands and there is not as yet a structured framework for implementation and evaluation. Among those that have been subject to scientific evaluation is the Matador programme described earlier (Box 6.2). Evaluations vary substantially, focusing on quality of care and processes, clinical outcomes and patient experience, or costs. Evaluations have been carried out by a range of organizations and groups, including the ZonMw, research institutes and universities (Pepels, Linden van der & Huijsman 2004, Steuten 2006). Funding agencies tend to emphasize cost–effectiveness. It has been suggested that a significant barrier to developing appropriate evaluation methods for chronic care programmes in the Netherlands has been the lack of an overall national vision and framework for such programmes (ZonMw 2006b). The Government encourages new diabetes care groups to report to the National Institute for Public Health and the Environment (RIVM) to inform the development of future health policies.

The RIVM and the Netherlands Institute for Health Services Research (NIVEL) regularly publish data on the incidence, prevalence and burden of chronic diseases, based on registrations in primary care and patient panels. However, there is little information about the relationship between health care settings and outcomes. NIVEL provides information on innovative programmes, including the types and contents of the programmes; but there is also little information on the performance of these programmes. It is thus not possible, at the time of writing, to clearly identify the impact of chronic care programmes on the overall performance of the Dutch health system in terms of efficiency, effectiveness, acceptability, accessibility and equity. While evaluations of individual programmes such as the Matador programme in the Maastricht region (Box 6.2) provide insights into some aspects, findings cannot be generalized for the entire country.

A key feature of disease management is the systematic use of appropriate management instruments at programme level and at the level of individual patient care. In the Dutch system, health professionals tend to be familiar with innovations at the individual patient level, but less so with organizational-level innovations. There is as yet little awareness that innovations should be integrated at both levels. The current nature of the primary care system, characterized by fragmentation, poses a challenge to those seeking to change attitudes among people working within the system.

ZonMw recently concluded that there is still fragmentation of chronic care in the Dutch health care system, suggesting a need for stronger leadership by the Government and recommending further research into the opportunities for chronic disease management (ZonMw 2006b). The Government is in the process of developing a framework for chronic disease management and encourages the development of diabetes programmes through diabetes care groups, described earlier. It recently formed a Task Group, chaired by a government-appointed physician; this group has formulated criteria, in the areas of quality of care, infrastructure, data collection and exchange (Hoogervorst 2005), which have to be met by diabetes care groups in order to qualify for subsidies.

Based on the experience with diabetes care groups, the Government intends to create an infrastructure for chronic care. It has become apparent that approaches differ: most groups are initiated by GPs, although others have been initiated by laboratories that contract with GPs. They organize laboratory tests, provide information to GPs and some employ specialist nurses to advise

> **Box 6.2 Evaluating the Matador programme**
>
> Evaluation is an essential management tool of the Matador programme. It uses benchmarking and feedback as well as annual reports to authorities, including the local health insurer. Patient focus groups were consulted to track patient experience and satisfaction throughout the programme. Patients are also asked to provide regular oral feedback about Matador.
>
> In 2004, the Matador programme was formally evaluated by ZonMw as part of a wider evaluation of the transmural care projects that it subsidized (ZonMw 2006a). The evaluation reported a range of successes achieved by the Matador programme, including improvement of diabetes care through the cooperation of 58 general practitioners (GPs), six endocrinologists and seven specialized diabetes nurses; identification of sources for structural financing; the introduction of new training opportunities for advanced clinical nurse specialists; low dropout rate; and the provision of care at the same cost as usual care.
>
> At the same time, it identified a number of failures, including the failure to develop an integrated electronic patient record system; a lack of communication between members of the core team, even though there was good cooperation; and sub-optimal patient self-management support.
>
> In a separate evaluation of the Matador programme, Steuten (2006) assessed clinical outcomes following the transformation of the programme from a transmural care project into a formal disease management programme (DMP) for patients with diabetes. She used a probabilistic decision model (Markov) to assess the long-term cost utility of Matador and the Maastricht Chronic Obstructive Pulmonary Disease (COPD)/asthma approach. Regarding diabetes care, she identified improvements in several outcome measures, including glycaemic control, health-related quality of life, patient adherence to treatment and certain behaviours. Further, she showed that the total costs of the programme allocated to medical specialists, specialized nurses and GPs did not change significantly, while there was a 54% decline in hospitalization costs in the group assigned to nurses, with an estimated saving of an average of €117 per patient per year and an increase in the level of health-related quality of life of 5% (Steuten et al. 2007).

and treat patients in cooperation with their GP. Diabetes care groups provide care according to the principles of a disease management programme and are obliged to collect benchmarking data, use feedback mechanisms and submit data to the NPCG, which is part of the NIVEL. The diabetes care groups use protocols based on nationally accepted guidelines, such as those developed by the Dutch College of General Practitioners.

Investing in the future

As noted earlier, health insurance in the Netherlands is privately run, but within a framework set out under public law. The 2006 Health Insurance Act aims to maintain the social character of the Dutch health care system, with health insurance accessible to all residents, regardless of their health status or social circumstances.

However, the Government has only indirect instruments through which to control insurers and providers. The Government and public depend heavily on the way insurers and providers interact and deliver care. Therefore, the Health Insurance Act can be seen not only as an opportunity to improve the quality of care, but also as a challenge to the principle of solidarity upon which the system is based (Table 6.1).

The new Health Insurance Act gives health insurers more freedom to secure services for their customers, based on an expectation that incentives for innovation may reduce health care expenditure. While the nominal premium that the insured have to pay to access the statutory package of essential services may not differ for those signing up to a particular insurance fund, insurers may compete on the quality of health care. This may prompt health insurers to become involved in the development of chronic disease management programmes. There is, however, a risk that health insurers may value cost-containment over quality of care. To ensure high quality of care, the Government will need to monitor developments through bodies such as the Health Inspectorate, which supervises health insurers and providers. Yet, this is likely to introduce another level of bureaucracy into the systems, without clear evidence that there will be any contribution to improved quality of health care delivery.

By introducing diabetes care groups, the Government intends to create a framework for stimulating regional health plans. The Dutch Health Care Authority (NzA) seeks to ensure that health plans can compete with each other. Thus, it is likely that the NzA will require providers to offer competing health plans within each region and to give enrolees real choice.

The 2006 Health Insurance Act was accompanied by a reform of the AWBZ in the form of the newly introduced Social Support Act (WMO), mentioned earlier. Through the WMO, municipalities have gained greater responsibility in the field of home care. While presenting an opportunity for local government to improve local care facilities for those in need, this has the potential to increase inequity in access to care.

The role of GPs is central to the Dutch health care system. They are the first point of contact for patients and act as gatekeepers. GPs monitor their patients through an electronic patient record system. However, those at primary and secondary care levels do not always cooperate well, reflecting differences in the type of care provided, organizational structures, financing arrangements, and systems of communication, as described earlier. Those working on both sides of the interface need to address these challenges.

There is growing support for a redesigned health care system, which shifts the focus from acute care to chronic and elderly care. This is demonstrated by the number of programmes being developed and implemented.

Table 6.1 *Chronic disease management in the Netherlands: strengths and weaknesses*

Strengths	Weaknesses	Opportunities	Threats
Health insurance system is of a private nature, with strong support under public law and solidarity	Lack of cooperation between primary and secondary care	Health Insurance Act: provides many opportunities to improve health care	Health Insurance Act: risk of undermining the principle of solidarity underlying health care
Role of the GP, strong gatekeeper function	Fragmented system of integrated care	Decentralization of the AWBZ: potential to improve health care by increasing responsibilities of local municipalities	Decentralization of the AWBZ: potential for increasing inequalities in access to care
Presence of electronic patient records in every GP practice	Lack of vision and strategy in the implementation of integrated care	Role of health insurers: involved in new types of care	Role of health insurers: reduced quality of health care due to focus on cost-efficiency
Growing awareness of need to change	Lack of available data due to lack of evaluation mechanisms	Development of strong vision and strategies towards the implementation of integrated care programmes	Pressure from lobby groups such as health professional groups
Support of the implementation of chronic disease management programmes	Lack of acceptance of authority	New roles of health professionals, especially nurses with potential to improve the quality of care	Continued shortage of nurses
	Lack of patient involvement	Guidelines for health professionals, such as multidisciplinary teams	Role of nurses remains badly defined
		Increased attention to health education and health support	Lack of adequately trained professionals

Source: Authors' own compilation.

Notes: GP: General practitioner; AWBZ: Exceptional Medical Expenses Act.

The "bottom-up" approach used in the implementation of these programmes has unfortunately contributed to fragmentation. It reflects a lack of government strategy on issues such as integrated care and chronic disease management. The Government has only a few instruments to support providers who are willing and able to take the lead in innovations.

The system in place at the time of writing is hampered by a lack of data, appropriate information and communication technology, and the evaluation tools necessary for effective management. There is a need to create a common framework for data collection and evaluation and to involve patients and their organizations in evaluation and further developments. Finally, there is a need to involve health professionals. The health care workforce is complex, with many roles and hierarchies. Coordinated care approaches create new roles for professionals, in particular the nursing profession. If implemented carefully, their involvement may improve the quality of care and reduce costs. However, as noted earlier, there is considerable resistance on the part of GPs and medical specialists to the idea of another professional group taking on their responsibilities and tasks. New roles can also be seen as a threat as they risk increasing future shortages of nurses. Thus, as nurses take on an even greater number of roles, tasks and responsibilities, basic tasks will have to be left to less-qualified personnel, who themselves require enhanced training. Multidisciplinary teams and cooperation across sectors should thus be encouraged: strong leadership from professionals in health care, insurers and government, together with a clear vision, will improve the chances of successful chronic care management.

References

DIEP (2008) [web site]. DIEP Diabetes Interactief Educatie Programma [DIEP Diabetes Interactive Education Programme]. Maastricht, DIEP Diabetes Interactief Educatie Programma (LifeScan, Johnson & Johnson) (http://www.diep.info/, accessed 22 August 2008).

Dutch Institute for Healthcare Improvement (2008) [web site]. CBO: 25 years of quality improvement. PLACE, Dutch Institute for Healthcare Improvement (http://www.cbo.nl/english/default_view, accessed 22 August 2008).

Eijkelberg IMJG et al. (2001). From shared care to disease management; key-influencing factors. *International Journal of Integrated Care*, 1:e17.

Hoogervorst H (2005). *Standpunt rapport taakgroep diabetes [Taskforce report on diabetes]*. The Hague, Ministry of Health, Welfare and Sport.

Kodner DL, Spreeuwenberg C (2002). Integrated care: meaning, logic, application: a discussion paper. *International Journal of Integrated Care,* 1:e12.

Linden B (2000). *The birth of integration, explorative studies on the development and implementation of integrated care in the Netherlands.* Dissertation. Utrecht, University of Utrecht.

Linden van der BA, Spreeuwenberg C, Schrijvers A (2001). Integration of care in the Netherlands: the development of transmural care since 1994. *Health Policy,* 55:111–120.

Maarse H (2006). Health insurance reform 2006. *Health Policy Monitor,* 3 (March).

Maastricht Transmural Diabetes Organisation (2000). *Matador protocol.* Maastricht, Maastricht Transmural Diabetes Organisation [unpublished].

Ministry of Health Welfare and Sport (2006). *Wet Maatschappelijke Ondersteuning. Iedereen moet mee kunnen doen [Act on Social Support, everybody should be able to participate].* The Hague, Netherlands Ministry of Health, Welfare and Sport.

Mur-Veeman I, Eijkelberg I, Spreeuwenberg C (2001). How to manage the implementation of shared care: a discussion of the role of power, culture and structure in the development of shared care arrangements. *Journal of Managed Medicine,* 15:142–155.

NPCG (2008) [web site]. Nationaal Panel Chronisch Zieken en Gehandicapten [National Panel for chronically ill people and handicapped persons] (http://www.nivel.nl/oc2/Page.asp?PageID=2232, accessed May 2008).

Pepels R, Van der Linden BA, Huijsman R (2004). *Vooral doen! Handreiking voor succesvol implementeren van transmurale zorg [A helping hand for successful implementation of transmural care].* Assen, Van Gorcum.

Spreeuwenberg C et al. (2000). *Handboek transmurale zorg [Handbook of transmural care].* Maarssen, Elsevier.

Steuten LMG et al. (2002). Participation of general practitioners in disease management: experiences from the Netherlands. *International Journal of Integrated Care,* 2:1 –7(e24).

Steuten LMG (2006). *Evaluation of disease management programmes for chronically ill.* Maastricht, Maastricht University.

Steuten LMG et al. (2007). A disease management programme for patients with diabetes mellitus is associated with improved quality of care within existing budgets. *Diabetic Medicine,* 24:1112–1120.

Vrijhoef HJM (2002). *Is it justifiable to treat chronic patients by nurse specialists? Evaluation of effects on quality of care*. Maastricht, Maastricht University.

Vrijhoef HJM et al. (2001). Adoption of disease management model for diabetes in region of Maastricht. *British Medical Journal,* 323:983–985.

ZonMw (2006a). *Successen van Matador-project samengevat [Successes of the Matador project]*. The Hague, ZonMw.

ZonMw (2006b). *Voorstel voor een Stimuleringsprogramma zorgverbetering chronisch zieken [Proposal for a programme to improve the health of the chronically ill]*. The Hague, ZonMw.

Chapter 7
Sweden

Ingvar Karlberg

Context

High-quality health care and equal access to services for all are the key goals of the Health and Medical Services Act adopted by the Swedish Parliament in 1982 (Glenngård et al. 2005). Under this Act, the 18 county councils, 2 regions and 290 municipalities in Sweden are responsible for the financing, organization and provision of health care and medical services, and for public health services for all residents who are entitled to use the services at subsidized prices.

The Swedish system is based on the Beveridge model, with counties and municipalities as providers of care; health care financing is predominantly through taxes at the regional and local levels. Taxes are proportional and there are no exemptions, with the 1998 law relating to priorities specifying that a person with acute needs should always be treated, regardless of the expected long-term outcome. A mandatory national-level social insurance system covers sick leave and pensions; it is funded through payroll taxes and administered by the State.

The counties are responsible for primary health care; they own, finance and run acute care hospitals, including psychiatric care. Municipalities are financially and organizationally responsible for the provision of all forms of nursing care for individuals above the age of 65, and also for chronic psychiatric care. Local taxes support all institutional and home care, although the individual receiving care is also required to make co-payments according to ability to pay. Any medical care provided in facilities operated by municipalities that requires physician consultation is the responsibility of the council, executed though the local primary health care centre (PHCC).

GPs employed by the county are generally responsible for a population defined by geographical boundaries; GPs operating in private practice contract with the county, with reimbursement based on capitation. District nurses, midwives, psychologists and physiotherapists are all licensed, work within health centres and are generally employed by the county. GPs have only limited gatekeeping functions and no financial incentives to reduce referral levels.

The county councils are grouped into six medical care regions to facilitate cooperation in tertiary care. Each region hosts one or two regional hospitals. The hospitals in Sweden are divided into district county hospitals, central county hospitals and regional hospitals, depending on their size and degree of specialization. There are a total of eight regional hospitals, of which seven are affiliated with a medical school and also function as research and teaching hospitals. Regional hospitals are owned and administered by the county in which they are located, supported by reimbursements from neighbouring county councils for care provided to their residents (regulated by agreements among the county councils within each region). The central Government provides compensation for the costs associated with teaching and research in these hospitals.

The State is generally not involved in directly financing health and social care; direct responsibility is limited to forensic medicine, prison health care and national defence, as well as services for refugees and immigrants who have not yet been admitted to a municipality. The Government has legal powers in matters of security, competence and accreditation of systems and equipment, and licensing of personnel. Although the financial viability of counties and municipalities is based on local taxation, state subsidies are common, with earmarked funding for areas that the central Government wishes to support.

Sweden has one of the oldest populations in the Organisation for Economic Co-operation and Development (OECD), along with Japan, France and Norway; however, the fraction of those aged 65 years and over is the highest among OECD countries. Expected survival at birth is at one of the highest levels in the world, an achievement driven by a combination of societal and individual public health measures, education and equitable access to health care. As a consequence, the care of older people with complex chronic, age-related conditions and transient, acute needs for care has become a key concern in the Swedish health system. Several recent developments have sought to address this challenge. Most relevant in this context have been the 1992 Care of the Elderly Reform and the 1995 reform of psychiatric care. These provide the legal basis for cooperation between providers, an essential requirement to optimize care for those with chronic health problems.

Chronic care was elevated to a higher level of priority by the Swedish Parliamentary Priorities Commission reporting, in 1995, on "Priorities in Health Care: Ethics, Economy, Implementation" (Swedish Parliamentary Priorities Commission 1995). It emphasized the role of chronic care in a way that had not explicitly been recognized before. A number of influential stakeholders joined this "movement", supporting a trend towards prioritization of chronic care. This has, however, not yet reached service provision at the level of the municipality to the same degree as at the county level, despite the importance of the municipality in the provision of care.

Analysing the response

Approaches to chronic disease management

In Sweden, the PHCC is the basis for all chronic care. There are over 1000 PHCCs across Sweden, financed by the counties, of which 80% are run by the counties and employ all staff working in the PHCCs. The remainder are operated by private providers, mostly in large chains (Praktikertjänst AB). In addition to, or integrated with PHCCs, there are some 7000 clinics for maternal and child health, district physiotherapy, rehabilitation and others. These are organized and run by nurses, midwives, physiotherapists and other health professionals, employed by the counties, with GPs acting as consultants (NBHW 2005a).

The majority of PHCCs operated by the counties employ a minimum of two doctors and several other categories of health care workers. All PHCCs run nurse-led clinics for diabetes and hypertension and some for allergy, asthma and COPD, psychiatry and heart failure. Some of the larger centres also provide nurse-led clinics for chronic neurological disorders. In contrast, "independent" PHCCs tend to be smaller, with only one or two doctors, one nurse and a secretary. These smaller PHCCs may have a clearly designated nurse-led clinic, although nurses may also see patients independently. Thus, nurse-led clinics are most common for diabetes care and mostly found in publicly run PHCCs. An increasing number of PHCCs are also establishing nurse-led clinics for other categories of patients.

Hospital departments for internal medicine have also established nurse-led clinics for diabetes, allergy, asthma, COPD and hypertension, as well as heart failure, chronic neurological conditions and renal failure. Some hospitals may offer nurse-led clinics for home oxygen treatment and other conditions or interventions, depending on local need and culture.

> **Box 7.1 Examples of typical care pathways for patients with diabetes, stroke, dementia and mental illness in Sweden**
>
> Children and young people with **diabetes** are generally treated by specialists at hospital clinics; however, adults with diabetes are seen in primary health care centres (PHCCs). In both settings, these are nurse-led clinics. Specialist clinics also involve dieticians. All diabetes care – irrespective of age – is provided according to national guidelines and insulin is fully subsidized. National guidelines and registries on diabetes care are developed and operated by the State (National Board of Health and Welfare, NBHW), the Swedish Society of Medicine and the counties, and are financed by the counties.
>
> For **stroke** patients, the chain of care is from ambulance transport to the emergency room at the nearest county hospital and to a stroke ward. After a thorough diagnostic assessment including a CT brain scan, pharmaceutical treatment and – sometimes – thrombolysis, rehabilitation begins. One third of patients are discharged within two weeks and transferred for rehabilitation at outpatient clinics in the community or in the primary care setting. There are clinical guidelines for stroke patients linking all elements of the care pathway.
>
> People with **dementia** are screened at the primary care level and generally seen at specialist clinics before diagnosis, according to clinical guidelines. Home care or nursing home care is provided by the community. Patients with chronic mental illness (of more than three months' duration) are cared for by communities in special housing and home care following the 1995 reform of psychiatric care.

The current setting for people with chronic conditions, especially older people, aims to link primary health care, hospital care and community care through "chains of care" or care pathways. An elderly patient with a chronic disease will typically be screened at the primary care centre; further assessment and plans for treatment will be developed in the specialist care setting at the local hospital, with rehabilitation provided at the community centre. Such a "chain of care" may be based on local agreements between providers, developed from national or regional clinical guidelines. Within PHCCs and hospital departments, clinical guidelines are generally used for all types of chronic disease management (Box 7.1).

All citizens for whom home health care is appropriate will receive such care, for a small charge. Responsibility for this is negotiated between counties and communities. About half of the counties provide home health care; for the remainder this has been taken over by the communities. Communities also run nursing homes for people over 65 years of age and services for all patients with chronic mental illness (Box 7.2). These are staffed by nurses, nurse assistants and social workers. Nursing homes may include physiotherapists and a rehabilitation unit. Palliative care teams from hospitals and/or PHCCs provide care for patients dying at home.

The allocation of tasks in the field of health and social care to the counties and communities is based on legally defined responsibilities; there are no disease-specific exemptions. Each care provider has a legal obligation, derived from the Health and Medical Services Act, to assess care systematically, although the method of evaluation is not defined. Provision is guided by regional and local guidelines (see later).

Within each county there are 5 to 50 municipalities or communities, which share a common organizational model for planning, development, research and negotiation with the county. In this way each county and its communities form a provider network. Counties and communities have political boards; the provider networks sit on those boards with politicians from the county and the communities, respectively. This regional cooperation between counties and communities plays an important role in political decisions regarding the allocation of responsibilities for different areas of care, such as rehabilitation of the elderly and people with chronic conditions. For example, a person who has been hospitalized and then requires further care at home or in a nursing home will be provided with such after-care as part of the responsibilities of the community. Disagreements on responsibility for care do arise, however, because of the high costs of some treatment or services involved, for example for equipment for home care.

Box 7.2 Reforming care for older people

The Care of the Elderly Reform in 1992 ("Ädel-reform") has been of utmost importance in the Swedish health and social care system (Andersson & Karlberg 2000). It aimed *"to provide municipalities with the organizational and financial preconditions to provide freedom of choice for the patient, security and integrity in health care and social services for the elderly and disabled"* (Andersson & Karlberg 2000). It transferred responsibility for financing and provision of care of the elderly and people with chronic mental disorders from the counties to the municipalities. It has been estimated that this transfer involved reallocating a total of 20% of financing and provision from county to municipality level. The main reason for the reform was a perceived over-medicalization of the care of elderly people in geriatric facilities and in nursing homes that were operated much like hospitals. Also, in many hospitals, as many as 20% of patients in internal medicine occupied beds despite not requiring acute hospital care; they remained in hospital because of a shortage of nursing home beds.

Transferring financial responsibilities from county to municipality level following the 1992 reform resulted in an almost immediate reduction of the number of "bed blockers", falling from approximately 15% in acute hospital care in 1990 to 6% in 1994 and subsequently stabilizing at a low level (Andersson & Karlberg 2000). The average length of stay also fell to four days for surgery and five days for internal medicine. For the counties this reform led to a reduction of the number of beds from 12 per 1000 in 1988 to 4 per 1000 in 1998. Also, municipalities established many new nursing homes, supported by state subsidies, as part of the reform.

> **Box 7.3 Nurse-led clinics in Sweden**
>
> The decision to establish a nurse-led clinic is generally made locally, at a hospital department or primary health care centre (PHCC). In reality, most clinics have developed from doctor–nurse cooperation into an independent nurse-led clinic. Another method by which nurse-led clinics are established is within the framework of a research project, usually a clinical study which requires a designated person (often a nurse) to be responsible for administration, registration, randomization, follow-up according to protocol and reporting. The staff involved will have acquired very special skills while working within the study and will be familiar with all the patients involved. It thus appears plausible to translate this experience into a routine nurse-led clinic. Examples include clinical studies on breast cancer and hypertension. Nurses in nurse-led clinics receive in-house training and they attend external courses and conferences. An increasing number also have academic affiliations and training.

Distribution, uptake and coverage

It is not possible to give a precise figure regarding the total number of nurse-led clinics in Sweden, although almost every medical department and PHCC has established such clinics (Box 7.3). The widespread availability of nurse-led clinics in the country is in part a reflection of financial considerations, based on the argument that assigning a nurse as a first point of contact to identify those who require a physician's care is more cost-effective than using a doctor in the first place. Nurse-led clinics are also considered a means to create new career opportunities for nurses and to develop a more client-oriented system for patients with chronic conditions and for elderly people with communication difficulties. Moreover, it has not been possible to recruit a sufficient number of doctors to meet the demand for health care in the Swedish system.

There are no significant regional differences in the number and design of nurse-led clinics; staffing depends on the catchment area. One or more diabetes nurses can be employed together with a dietician, a podiatrist, a surgeon and a diabetes physician or endocrinologist. As noted earlier, all citizens are fully covered by counties and communities and have access to all available programmes and care networks. All citizens are treated according to need, without exemption.

A patient journey: Sweden

As noted earlier, in Sweden primary care is the first point of contact for patients with chronic disease and the last point of referral once patients have been seen at specialist clinics. Generally, specialist clinics do not see chronic patients again after the first assessment, or only during an annual follow-up visit; the PHCC and district nurses provide the basic day-to-day provision, including prescriptions and paperwork for social and technical support. Hospital care is generally temporary and only for acute treatment. Patients in Sweden have to pay for family medicine – primary care, however, and referral from the PHCC to all other services, are free. Patients who do not have a referral will have to pay for secondary care provided in hospital or at a specialized clinic; this policy aims to incentivize utilization of the PHCC and so reduce use of hospital clinics. In addition, a system of (capped) regressive co-payment exists for medication.

In Sweden a hypothetical patient (described here) would pursue the care pathway set out in the following paragraphs. The patient is a 54-year-old woman with type 2 diabetes and COPD who has a leg ulcer and moderate retinopathy. She is also moderately obese (BMI of 27), has been unemployed for three years, receives social assistance benefits and lives on her own.

If this patient is a local resident, she will most likely be registered at the PHCC and the department of internal medicine at the nearest hospital. She will be a patient at the nurse-led clinics at both sites and will be referred to the relevant specialist, when appropriate, as determined by the nurse, or upon request by the patient or her relatives. The patient will only visit the hospital-based physician in the event of sudden deterioration of her condition or for a new assessment. The treatment recommended by the specialist will be carried out mainly at the PHCC. She may have one or two follow-up visits to the hospital clinic as well as an annual check-up.

Self-care will always be encouraged, particularly at nurse-led clinics and by the dietician. The nurses at both sites will have regular contact with the district nurse, as well as home health care services when required. Home health care is either the responsibility of primary care within the county, or a community responsibility, with the exception of GP activities; these will always be a county responsibility, as previously described. Home care is part of the social system within the community, and is a patient right, although it does require co-payment.

The provision of technical devices and support for disabled people and people with chronic conditions is mainly a community responsibility. However, the boundary between county and community responsibility in this sector is not clear and is often subject to negotiations.

Health system features supporting programmes

Targets, standards and guidelines

As noted earlier, provision of care in Sweden is generally steered by guidelines and protocols. Sweden operates an elaborate system of prospective disease registries, at present covering over 50 diseases. Registries are operated by the counties, include individual patient data, and are used for quality assessment

> **Box 7.4 Regional oncology centres in Sweden**
>
> The Swedish Cancer Registry started in 1958 with the National Board of Health and Welfare (NBHW) responsible for storing and analysing data collected directly from each hospital or each county. During the 1970s, Regional Cancer Centres were introduced, financed partly by the State and partly by the counties. Each region has had its own Regional Cancer Centre since 1982. Regional Cancer Centres have three main responsibilities: (1) collecting and analysing cancer data, and reporting to the national registry; (2) developing clinical guidelines to encourage cost-effective care and to ensure equality between providers within the country (this is the most developed area of "disease management" in the Swedish health system); and (3) monitoring cancer care in quality registries so as to enable boards, professional groups and managers of each Regional Cancer Centre, the regional authority and local hospitals to observe the extent to which established guidelines are being adhered to.
>
> Each set of clinical guidelines is reviewed by professional, administrative, financing and political bodies, all of whom have been collaborating for a long time, thereby developing common language, common ideologies and, ultimately, a common culture. In addition, some areas where medical outcomes were poor in the 1970s have been much improved through national multi-centre research governed and organized jointly by the Regional Cancer Centres.

and quality improvement. Registry data are used by the National Board of Health and Welfare (NBHW) to develop evidence-based national guidelines, further informed by evidence compiled by the Swedish Council of Technology Assessment in Health Care. National guidelines are generally translated into local programmes; they are designed to improve quality of care, ensure equity in treatment methods and indications for treatment, as well as equitable access to care, and to contain costs.

There are registries and national guidelines for diabetes, coronary heart disease, renal failure, hip fracture and hip replacement, cataract surgery, stroke and all forms of cancer (Box 7.4). The development of regional and local clinical guidelines, often based on national guidelines, is encouraged by all counties and communities.

Examples of guidelines for specific diseases are:

- Every county, hospital and PHCC has developed guidelines and programmes for diabetes. Increasingly, patient self-management and the need for change of lifestyle is included in patient education.

- Research on stroke has indicated that organizational factors and skill levels are important in achieving good outcomes. In addition, medical treatment, with rapid diagnostic scans and use of thrombolysis, is expanding. Stroke is increasingly seen as an emergency, with urgent medical needs similar to myocardial infarction.

> **Box 7.5 Care for those with mental illness**
>
> Psychiatric care in Sweden is generally seen as insufficient at both community and council levels, largely because of a shortage of personnel, in particular doctors. The Government has implemented several measures to improve mental health care, such as national assessments, guidelines, improved education and earmarked funding. Yet, 10 years after the 1995 reform of psychiatric care, many communities have not been able to establish all elements of good mental health care, rehabilitation and supported employment. Many projects are testing new approaches in community-based mental health care, often aiming at integrating county and community care with rehabilitation and employment. Yet, few results have been implemented into clinical practice.
>
> The number of hospitals beds for psychiatric care is 360 per million population (or 3000 in the entire country). Counties provide acute psychiatric care in county hospitals and outpatient care at specialist clinics. It is expected that almost all voluntary treatment will be provided in outpatient clinics and primary care.

- Guidelines for care of patients with dementia are in place in most counties and communities, and more are being developed. A newly published overview by the Swedish Council of Technology Assessment in Health Care will be important for the future development of dementia care (Swedish Council on Technology Assessment in Health Care 2008a, Swedish Council on Technology Assessment in Health Care 2008b).
- Care for patients with mental illness is an underdeveloped medical area in which the central Government has actively stimulated regional and local developments. The area is still bearing the consequences of the 1995 reform of psychiatric care which transferred responsibility for long-term mental care to the communities (Box 7.5).

National guidelines normally do not include any specific guidance on the organization of local care (as, for example, in nurse-led clinics) since the responsibility for organization and financing of care rests with the counties. However, there are legal restrictions on the nature and scope of activities and interventions performed by registered nurses.

Evaluation and lessons learned

As noted earlier, the 1992 Care of the Elderly Reform and the 1995 reform of psychiatric care transferred responsibility for a large part of health care for the elderly and for people with chronic conditions to the municipalities. This represented a considerable paradigm change, since pre-1992 municipalities only had to comply with the social legislation, whereas from 1992 they have to meet the requirements of two very different sets of legal principles: the Health and Medical Services Act, giving municipalities the legal duty to provide for care, while social legislation stipulates formal rights for clients.

This legislation clarifies the roles and responsibilities of counties and municipalities in the field of health and social care and, in essence, forms the basis for cooperation and coordination. Thus, municipalities have full responsibility for care and social support of patients over the age of 65 years who have chronic health problems; however, any medical support through family doctors is not part of municipalities' remit, as provision of the latter is the responsibility of the county council. Cooperation is thus necessary to enhance care for those with complex needs. Coordination and/or cooperation are often more developed in rural settings than in urban settings.

Each county and community has a right, and indeed an obligation, to conduct research and development projects and there are several hundred projects currently ongoing related to the care and support of patients with chronic disease(s). Most of these are not disease specific, but focus instead on the health and social care structure.

More recently there has been a trend, at the county level, towards a more formal development of local coordination (*närsjukvård*) and all counties are developing strategic plans for local coordination to strengthen the links between providers. In 2005 the NBHW presented a report on local coordination, which showed that there is no common, national solution to better coordination; instead, approaches tend to be tailored to local needs (NBHW 2005b). Primary health care is usually at the core, with municipality care on one side and hospital or specialized care on the other. In several counties, this *närsjukvård* has strengthened primary health care, sometimes reinforced by one or more specialists making regular visits, and working groups involving the community. The main focus is on the elderly and on people with multiple chronic diseases, including mental disabilities. Rehabilitation units and mental health care units are of special interest for people with chronic conditions.

By 2002, most county councils had established at least one "chain of care" or care pathway, as described earlier. The majority of chains of care are designed around patients with chronic conditions. Improving the quality of care was reported to be the major drive behind most initiatives and, although success has been mixed, there seems to be strong motivation at the county council level to continue and to further develop chains of care (Åhgren 2003).

These two developments, chains of care and local coordination (*närsjukvård*) are running in parallel, and at many sites and/or in many disease areas, they have been merged.

Given the strong decentralization of the Swedish health care system, and the autonomy of the counties, there is a risk of regional inequality in the development of and access to chains of care and/or *närsjukvård*. However, there is an expectation that the newly formed national Swedish Association of Local Authorities and Regions (SALAR) may facilitate enhanced integration at the local level. The SALAR was formed in 2007 by a merger of the Swedish Association of Local Authorities (SALA) and the Federation of Swedish County Councils (FCC); it represents the governmental, professional and employer-related interests of Sweden's municipality and county councils (SALAR 2007). The formation of the SALAR is also expected to have a significant impact on the choice of areas for development of guidelines and the organizational and financial impact of any such guidelines. The NBHW has a role in facilitating cooperation on medical matters between the new body and the State. Together, they will address both medical and social sector legislation, financing, programmes and activities.

Investing in the future

Chronic disease management is a major part of health care in Sweden, as reflected in the volume of initiatives directed at access and service development. Organizational change is adapting to the effects of compression of morbidity. Medical developments are increasingly directed towards patients needing chronic care and their families, with capacity increasing in particular for care and support to people with dementia, osteoporosis, cataract(s), heart failure, incontinence and cancer. A remaining weak point is the lack of cooperation and communication between providers, that is, between counties and municipalities, and in the "triangle" linking primary care, hospital care and community care, as noted earlier. However, new legislation and projects designed to foster a higher degree of integration are currently being developed.

Several further issues related to chronic disease management in Sweden remain (Table 7.1). Thus, the legal status of primary care physicians in community care will probably not easily be changed. A pilot project gave five communities the legal right to run primary health care services; however, after five years the project was terminated as the results did not support further development in that direction. The social paradigm characterizing community provision of support seemed incompatible with the medical culture in primary care.

At the local level, an increasing degree of integration between different providers can be observed. However, there are no signs as yet indicating major changes in chains of responsibility.

Other obstacles are purely technical. Thus, electronic communication systems are not compatible between hospitals and PHCCs, between PHCCs and communities and between counties. There are no national technical norms or criteria for IT systems in health care; this is left to the relevant local authority,

Table 7.1 *Chronic disease management in Sweden: strengths and weaknesses*

Strengths	Weaknesses	Opportunities	Threats
Clear and sustainable framework set by 1982 Health Act, the 1992 Care of the Elderly Reform and the 1995 reform of psychiatric care. No major changes suggested by political parties on either side	Tax financing always subject to political priorities	Interest in cooperation between providers is increasing at local and regional levels. Seamless care is considered less expensive and service quality has become more important as a result of demands from families and children born in the 1940s and 1950s	Insufficient national financial development to support health care at the current level
	Elected political representatives on management boards: political management with insufficient management skills		Changing demography with an increasing proportion of older people (18% over age 65 in 2006 (projected for 2020: 25%) with higher need levels; main challenges in the area of dementia
Simple and clear financing principles; taxes and minor co-payments for health care set according to personal resources for community care	Cooperation between providers within counties and between county and community care is not functioning well, particularly in urban centres	National legal restrictions are less strict, providing more opportunities for local solutions	Lack of personnel due to decreasing interest in the health care sector, and in competition with industry, increasing wages
Access to care and provision of care generally considered equitable; however the large number of providers inevitably leads to inequities. Politically this is also seen as a strength, adjusting provision to the local needs	Cooperation between providers of long-term care and rehabilitation of individuals with mental illness-related disabilities is highly criticized	Centralization of policy decisions by politicians in counties has reduced the level of political management at production level	

(cont.)

Table 7.1 *(cont.)*

Strengths	Weaknesses	Opportunities	Threats
High educational level of personnel, with academic training for almost all groups	Relative lack of incentives in care produced by public providers leads to low productivity. In combination with heavy demands, this leads to poor access in some medical areas, along with waiting lists	Increased interest among politicians and top managers in evaluation and assessment of production both in terms of service (access) and results (outcome)	Poor access leads to an increasing number of people purchasing private insurance: this may lead to decreased interest in financing universal care through taxes
Unrestricted access to unplanned and acute care			
Community care is generally of high quality, with new infrastructure and well-trained personnel	Free access to accident and emergency services leads to long waiting times	Increased interest in academic training and scientific methods, not only in terms of medical activities but also in management	Insufficient access to long-term care and special housing (nursing homes), and lack of integration between providers, potentially leading to individuals opting for private providers; this may undermine the tax basis for public provision and contribute to inequality between socioeconomic groups
	Shortage of GPs in primary care and of specialists in psychiatry	More academic influence on personnel training; shift of generations is improving skills, competencies and changing culture in the care sector	
	Lack of personnel for clients in nursing homes		
	Domestic care (provided to 10% above age 65) is believed to be impersonal		

Source: Authors' own compilation.

Note: GP: General practitioner.

which has a legal obligation to issue a tender and to purchase the cheapest product. It has only been possible in two counties to implement the same system in hospital care and at PHCCs (*vårdadministrativt system* in Norbotten and Halland (Halland County Council 2007)). A national project is currently being developed to extract information from patients' records at all provider levels, based on the personal identification number (PIN). This is still in the first phase of development; however, it is controversial, as some political parties oppose national registries based on the PIN due to the potential violation of confidentiality.

Numerous projects are also aiming to improve the care of elderly people, in mental health care and in the field of chronic disease(s). A few are trying to integrate different systems, such as health care, social care and employment for patients with psychiatric disabilities. Most projects appear to be initiated by individuals. Funding varies, with most being research and development projects that are locally financed (Möller 2005). Few have scientific significance and are translated into action.

A state commission is currently examining the regional organization of state agencies and the role of state governance. Several state agencies have geographical boundaries that are not congruent with those of regional authorities. The commission is seeking to coordinate these boundaries, in a process that will eventually lead to significant changes in health care organization.

There is no ongoing comprehensive assessment of the system for provision and financing of health care. In 1999 the Committee on Funding and Organization of Health Care ("HSU 2000"), appointed by the Government in 1992, presented a report on alternative mechanisms for financing (taxes, insurance, other) and organization (to reduce tiers of administration within the Swedish system) (Socialdepartementet 1999). This exercise was repeated subsequently; however, the system itself appears to be resistant to major change.

In its recent report, the National Coordinator on Psychiatry proposed state grants to communities in order to improve competences and skills among community staff working in long-term mental health care, as well as some resources to improve integration with other providers (Socialdepartementet 2006). This report was delivered to the Government by the Ministry of Social Affairs and has led to limited additional support by the Government, mainly for developmental projects.

References

Åhgren B (2003). Chain of care development in Sweden: results of a national study. *International Journal of Integrated Care*, 3:e01.

Andersson G, Karlberg I (2000). Integrated care for the elderly: the background and effects of the reform of Swedish care of the elderly. *International Journal of Integrated Care*, 1(1):1–10.

Glenngård A et al. (2005). Health systems in transition: Sweden. *Health Systems in Transition*, 7(4):1–128.

Halland County Council (2007) [web site]. Welcome to the Halland County Council. Halmstad, Halland County Council (http://www.lthalland.se/lth_templates/informationpage____1406.aspx, accessed 22 August 2008).

Möller P (2005). *Forskning och utveckling i kommuner, landsting och regioner [Research and development in municipalities, county councils and regions]*. Stockholm, Sveriges Kommuner och Landsting.

NBHW [National Board of Health and Welfare] (2005a). *Hälso- och sjukvårdsrapport [Health care report]*. Stockholm, Socialstyelsen.

NBHW [National Board of Health and Welfare] (2005b). *Nationell handlingsplan för hälso- och sjukvården [National action plan for health care]*. Stockholm, Socialstyelsen.

Socialdepartementet (2006). *Slutbetänkande av Nationell psykiatrisamordning, Ambition och ansvar. Nationell strategi för utveckling av amhällets insatser till personer med psykiska sjukdomar och funktionshinder [Final report by the national psychiatry coordination, ambition and responsibility. National strategy for the development of societal efforts for individuals with mental disease and disability]*. Stockholm, Socialdepartementet.

Socialdepartementet (1999). *HSU 2000, God vård på lika villkor? Om statens styrning av hälso – och sjukvården [Good care on equal conditions? About the State's control of health care]*. Stockholm, Socialdepartementet.

SALAR (2007) [web site]. About SALAR. Stockholm, Swedish Association of Local Authorities and Regions (http://www.skl.se/artikel.asp?C=6392&A=48652, accessed 22 August 2008).

Swedish Council on Technology Assessment in Health Care (2008a). *Dementia – Etiology and epidemiology. A systematic review. Volume 1*. Stockholm, Swedish Council on Technology Assessment in Health Care.

Swedish Council on Technology Assessment in Health Care (2008b). *Dementia – Diagnostic and therapeutic interventions. A systematic review. Volume 2*. Stockholm, Swedish Council on Technology Assessment in Health Care.

Swedish Parliamentary Priorities Commission (1995). *Priorities in health care ethics, economy, implementation*. Stockholm, Regeringskansliets Offsetcentral.

Chapter 8
Australia

Nicholas Glasgow, Nicholas Zwar, Mark Harris,
Iqbal Hasan, Tanisha Jowsey

Context

The health system in Australia comprises "a mixture of public and private sector health service providers and a range of funding and regulatory mechanisms" (Australian Government Medicare Australia 2006a), providing universal access to health care for communities spread over vast geographical distances. There is no single funder or statutory body tasked with coordinating the provision of primary and secondary care in this system where both profit-making and non-profit-making organizations deliver health care.

The Commonwealth (federal) Government establishes national policies, sets the regulatory framework and provides funding through Medicare (Australian Government Medicare Australia 2006a), which encompasses the Medicare Benefits Schedule (MBS), the Pharmaceutical Benefits Scheme (PBS) and free access to public hospitals. It also provides a 30% rebate on private health insurance subscriptions. Medicare provides universal coverage for citizens, permanent residents, and visitors from countries with reciprocal arrangements with Australia. The MBS funds private doctors, including GPs, the majority of whom work in small private businesses, on a fee-for-service basis. It also provides some funding for practice nurses, psychologists and allied health professionals working in community settings. It includes some "pay for performance" items to reward quality in general practice and chronic disease management. The Commonwealth Government also provides specific funding for Aboriginal and Torres Strait Islander Health Services, residential aged care and a suite of programmes aimed specifically at addressing the challenges presented in delivering health services to rural and remote communities. These include the Rural Primary Health Programme, Multipurpose Services and the Royal Flying Doctors Service (Australian Government Department of Health and Ageing 2006a).

State and Territory governments are principally responsible for the provision of health services, including public health services, acute health services and a number of community-based services such as community nursing, allied health and public dental and mental health services. They maintain direct relationships with most health care providers, including regulation of health professionals and private hospitals.

Chronic disease has been a prominent focus for health system reform in Australia since the early 1990s. Interest has been provoked by national and international reports (such as the Australian Institute of Health and Welfare (AIHW) (Australian Institute of Health and Welfare 2006), data from the Australian Bureau of Statistics (ABS) (ABS 2007) and recommendations from the World Health Organization (WHO) (WHO 1981)), together with inputs from various government and public health departments. In some cases additional impetus has been provided by clinicians with particular concerns and by interest groups representing patients.

The degree to which reforms are coordinated across government varies, reflecting the division of responsibilities within the federal system. Examples of predominantly state-run programmes include the New South Wales (NSW) Health Chronic Disease Programme (Scott 2002) and the Primary Care Partnerships Strategy in Victoria (State Government of Victoria Department of Human Services 2006). The National Primary Care Collaborative (NPCC) programme (APCC 2006) is an example of a programme driven primarily by the Commonwealth Government.

Cooperation between the Commonwealth, Territory and State governments is facilitated by the intergovernmental Council of Australian Governments (COAG). Under its auspices, the Australian Health Ministers Conference (AHMC) meets to coordinate health policy, advised by the Australian Health Ministers Advisory Council (AHMAC). The AHMAC, composed of heads of health authorities of the Commonwealth and State governments, has an important role in driving the process that developed the National Health Priority Areas (Australian Government Department of Health and Ageing 2007a) and also supported the 2005 National Chronic Disease Strategy (NCDS) (National Health Priority Action Council 2005).

In 2006 the COAG committed funding of AUD 660 million (€400 million) from the Commonwealth and AUD 480 million (€290 million) from the States and Territories to the COAG "Better Health for all Australians" package that included two major policy directions relevant to chronic disease: the Australian Better Health Initiative (ABHI), with AUD 500 million (€305 million) (COAG 2006a); and the National Action Plan on Mental Health (COAG 2006b). The National Action Plan on Mental Health involves funding of a total of AUD 4.0 billion (€2.4 billion) across jurisdictions over five years.

The NCDS now provides the overarching direction for chronic disease prevention and care in Australia (National Health Priority Action Council 2005), with the ABHI and National Action Plan on Mental Health providing substantial resources to implement additional policies relevant to chronic disease. The NCDS focuses on improved prevention and better management of the major contributors to the chronic disease burden, driven by a broader agenda, at federal government level. While seeking to improve quality, State governments have a particular interest in decreasing the use of expensive hospital resources, reducing admissions, readmissions and length of stay. Health expenditure in some states, such as NSW, is increasing in real terms by up to 8% per annum, a level seen as unsustainable in the long term (NSW Government Treasury 2007).

Analysing the response

Approaches to chronic disease management

Coordinated, multidisciplinary care has been a major goal of Australian primary care since the 1990s, with trials of coordinated care leading to the introduction of multidisciplinary care plans within the 1999 Enhanced Primary Care (EPC) package. These initiatives drew on the Chronic Care Model (CCM) developed in the United States (Wagner, Austin & Von Korff 1996) and provide a mechanism for securing greater involvement by GPs, practice nurses and allied health professionals in structured and coordinated care. The EPC package included three programmes aimed at supporting chronic care:

(1) MBS items, allowing payments for annual health assessments for older people and for multidisciplinary care planning and case conferencing;

(2) a programme to educate GPs, allied health providers and the community about the EPC matters; and

(3) Commonwealth Carelink Centres to provide easier access to information.

GPs have, however, experienced difficulties in taking advantage of these developments, citing constraints relating to time, organization, communication, education and resources (Blakeman et al. 2001). In July 2005 the MBS care planning items were supplemented with the "General Practitioner Management Plan" (GPMP), which supports care planning by GPs, while the "Team Care Arrangement" (TCA) funds multidisciplinary support (Box 8.1).

There have been important changes in payment methods for chronic disease care, with an increasing move from fee-for-service payments to payment for performance. This is exemplified by incentives to improve care in general practice settings through the Practice Incentives Program (PIP) and Service Incentives Payments (SIP) programmes (Australian Government Medicare Australia 2008). These pay general practices contingent on their achievement of specified quality and service criteria. For example, the Diabetes SIP (described later) provides payment to practices for each patient completing an annual cycle of care (which includes assessment of HbA1c, blood pressure, lipids, weight, behavioural risk factors and screening for complications).

As noted earlier, there are also incentives for GPs to complete a care plan for patients with chronic disease and complex needs. Completion of a TCA within the EPC package generates a separate payment (which is more than fee-for-service payments for standard consultations). It also allows them to refer the patient to private allied health services (physiotherapy, psychologist, dietician, exercise physiologist, podiatrist, etc.) up to five times in each 12-month period. However, these additional (performance-based) payments make up less than 10% of GPs' incomes and they are not linked to outcome targets.

The EPC package further includes an element of self-management, in the Sharing Health Care Initiative (Australian Government Department of Health and Ageing 2005). This funded 12 demonstration projects, with further investment in self-management planned as part of the ABHI. It will provide training for health professionals to teach self-management skills.

All states have developed chronic disease self-management programmes (CDSMP). It is difficult to assess how widely these have been implemented within states or how well they have been sustained once the initial Commonwealth-funded programmes concluded. The 2006–2007 federal budget made a major investment (including matching funding from the states) in health promotion and early intervention with AUD 515 million (€310 million) allocated over five years. Self-management is one of the key programmes included in this initiative. It has been pointed out that integration of self-management activities into primary care will be important to the success of this initiative (Jordan & Osbourne 2007). While there have been some attempts to develop peer support groups and programmes, these have not been as well resourced as in some other countries (such as the Expert Patient Programme in the United Kingdom) and are seen as not having taken adequate account of the needs of people from culturally and linguistically diverse (CALD) backgrounds (Williams et al. 2007).

Box 8.1 Organization and financing of care planning

The General Practitioner Management Plan (GPMP) and Team Care Arrangement (TCA) within the revised Enhanced Primary Care (EPC) package aim to facilitate enhanced access to multidisciplinary care, including psychological services. Patients with chronic conditions and complex needs being managed with a care plan can receive a Medicare rebate for up to five allied health services per year, thereby expanding potential access to these services for those with low incomes. It also increases the involvement of allied health professionals in private practice in the care of chronic disease, for example by providing services such as podiatry for which there are long waiting times and limited service availability through the public system. Care plans thus present a change in the delivery system, as they offer a mechanism for funding a change in the role of the general practitioners (GPs) to encourage greater involvement in structured and coordinated care. In many general practices nurses assist substantially with development of care plans. This reduces the time taken to prepare the plan but the GP can still claim the full rebate so the process of nurse involvement is therefore a financial benefit to the practice. The level of the Medicare rebate for a GPMP is currently AUD 93.75 (€56) and a TCA is AUD 74.25 (€45).

According to standards developed by the Royal Australian College of General Practitioners (RACGP 2000) to support care planning, a multidisciplinary care plan should identify the patient's diagnosis, problems and needs, establish goals and tasks and liaise with a least two other providers. Yet the extent to which these different elements have been documented varies. For example, an audit study of 230 care plans for patients with type 2 diabetes (Vagholkar et al. 2007) found that while the majority of care plans listed two or more care providers (94%), just of half of the plans (57%) listed the patient's diagnosis, 32% their problems and 77% their needs, while 59% and 36% of plans, respectively, documented established goals and tasks. The content of the care plans was influenced by the type of template used and documented information was limited. The reasons for this are likely to be multiple and include time pressures faced by GPs.

In addition to the financial scheme introduced through the EPC package, the Australian Government has committed funding to the NPCC programme mentioned earlier (APCC 2006). Introduced in 2004, the NPCC aims to improve access, service delivery and integration of care for patients with complex and chronic conditions. The first of the planned three waves focused on diabetes care and secondary prevention of coronary heart disease. The approach relied on local activity in practices based on plan–do–study–act cycles. A total of 157 practices were involved in the first wave, which yielded demonstrable improvements in quality of care for patients with coronary heart disease (Farmer, Knight & Ford 2005). The second wave of the programme, known as the Australian Primary Care Collaboratives (APCC) has recently been launched, to run over four years starting from 2007–2008 (APCC 2006).

Approaches to chronic disease management in Australia have tended to focus on delivery system design and self-management support. Other elements of the CCM have received less attention so far, with the possible exception of decision support. For example, bodies such as the Royal Australian College of General

Practitioners (RACGP), the National Asthma Council, the National Heart Foundation and Diabetes Australia have produced clinical practice guidelines. Dissemination of guidelines is typically by mail, with a web-based version also available, but there has been very little support for active implementation or evaluation of uptake.

The Commonwealth Government's HealthConnect initiative has invested substantially in creating standards for e-health and conducting trials of e-health initiatives, such as shared electronic health records (Australian Government Department of Health and Ageing 2006b). Yet clinical information systems remain relatively underdeveloped. The most notable exception is the system for diabetes care mentioned earlier, where there are incentives for GPs to establish a disease register, which allows them to claim for a cycle of care on an annual basis.

In addition to the care planning and coordination schemes introduced through the EPC package, as an example of a generalist programme supporting any chronic illness of greater duration than six months, additional incentive schemes within the Medicare Benefits Schedule that target specific chronic diseases were introduced from 2001. For example, the Australian Asthma Management Plan (Woolcock et al. 1989, National Asthma Council Australia 2002) encompassed the Asthma 3+ Visit Plan. It provided payment on completion of a series of planned visits by patients with moderate to severe asthma. Consultations included assessment of severity, review of asthma-related medication, provision of a written asthma action plan, and education of the patient. This programme has now been replaced by the Asthma Cycle of Care. Evaluation of this programme and the resulting policy responses are discussed later, as is the National Integrated Diabetes Programme (NIDP).

The Better Outcomes in Mental Health initiative was introduced in the 2001–2002 budget. It has a number of components, including provision of education to GPs. Divisions of General Practice act as fundholders and provide access to psychology services.

Specific programmes have been developed for Aboriginal and Torres Strait Islanders including coordinated care trials involving improved care coordination, fund pooling, and some limited additional resources (Box 8.2). Aboriginal Community Controlled Health Services have specifically targeted chronic disease in their programmes. More information on these initiatives is available on the government-funded Indigenous Health Infonet web site (Australian Indigenous Health Infonet 2007). Other programmes focusing on the needs of Aboriginal and Torres Strait Islanders include the New South Wales Aboriginal vascular health programme (Scott 2002) and a number of State and Territory programmes tackling renal disease. In remote areas, geographical isolation and limited workforce capacity have impeded progress.

> **Box 8.2 Aboriginal and Torres Strait Islanders initiatives**
>
> There are two important national initiatives, developed in response to the early onset and high prevalence of chronic conditions in Aboriginal and Torres Strait Islander people (ABS 2005): the Adult Health Check and the Healthy for Life Programme.
>
> The Adult Health Check involves a new Medicare Benefit Schedule (MBS) item, introduced in 2004, to support preventive health assessments for Aboriginal and Torres Strait Islanders aged 15 to 54 years (Australian Government Department of Health and Ageing 2007b). This followed the introduction of a similar rebate for elderly people (over 74 years) in the general Australian population. However, the implementation of the initiative faced a number of challenges across the diverse primary health care settings where preventive assessments might be conducted, including limited access to medical practitioners in remote communities (Australian Institute of Health and Welfare 2001); the failure to identify Aboriginal or Torres Strait Islanders; limited awareness and experience of many general practitioners (GPs) providing care for this population (Britt et al. 2002); and slow uptake of the rebate by medical practitioners. Together, these challenges led to calls for greater financing of an appropriate implementation strategy (Mayers & Couzos 2004).
>
> The Commonwealth Healthy for Life Programme is designed to support quality improvement of maternal and child care and prevention and management of chronic illness in adults (Australian Government Department of Health and Ageing 2006c). The programme builds on research (Bailie et al. 2007, Si et al. 2005), documented experience and pilot projects of quality improvement interventions in Indigenous Australian settings (Australian Government Department of Health and Ageing 2006c) and is being implemented in primary health care services serving over 80 Aboriginal and Torres Strait Islander communities. These services are required to assess the state of service delivery, develop and implement action plans, and monitor service delivery and health outcomes through ongoing quality improvement cycles. The programme is at an early stage of implementation and is supported by a resource package; a panel of facilitators and a service toolkit (Australian Government Department of Health and Ageing 2006c). While the quality improvement approach is expected to enhance capacity significantly in chronic illness care it will be some years before the impact on service delivery and health outcomes becomes apparent.

Distribution, uptake and coverage

Chronic care programmes are provided in primary care settings, particularly in general practice locations and hospital outreach settings. State-funded and state-administered community health services also contribute to chronic disease care.

General practice programmes are organized and supported by Divisions of General Practice, typically in collaboration with public health services or, sometimes, with networks of private providers. In a 2004–2005 survey of Divisions of General Practice, all Divisions had at least one programme with a generic or specific focus on chronic disease (Hordacre et al. 2006). The most common programme areas were mental health (98% of Divisions) and diabetes (96% of Divisions). Fig. 8.1 shows the proportion of Divisions with chronic disease-focused programmes or activities.

Fig. 8.1 *Divisions of General Practice with chronic disease-focused programmes or activities, 2002–2003 to 2004–2005*

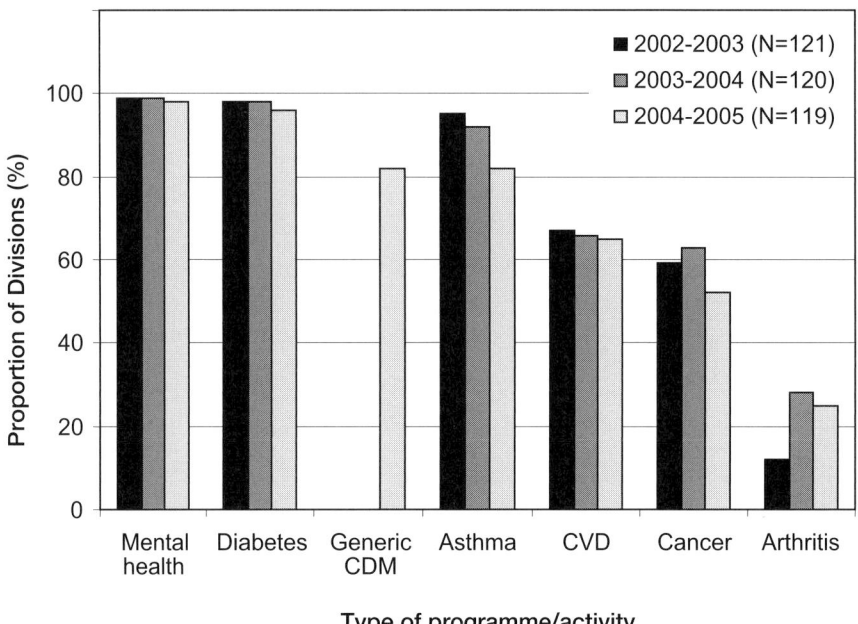

Source: Adapted from Hordacre et al. 2006.

Notes: CDM: Chronic disease management; *CVD:* Cardiovascular disease.

State Health Departments have developed a number of chronic disease initiatives which aim to reduce the burden of chronic disease and, in particular, their impact on hospitalization. Programmes focused on patients with cardiac failure and COPD are the most widespread, involving liaison nurses carrying out patients' post-discharge follow-up and linking with community-based services. Table 8.1 summarizes examples of state-based programmes.

Community health workers contributing to chronic disease care include primary health nurses, allied health professionals and mental health workers. As these professionals are employed by state health services and are located in community health centres or in hospitals, they need to work across organizational and geographic boundaries in order to collaborate with general practice staff.

GPs have been the professional group most intensely involved in the various chronic disease care initiatives in Australia. Their involvement can be judged

Table 8.1 *Chronic disease management programmes and strategies across states*

Strategy	Victoria	South Australia	Western Australia	Queensland	New South Wales	Tasmania
Establishment of regional structures to coordinate chronic disease initiatives	✓	✓			✓	✓
Outreach programmes to prevent readmission of patients with CHF to hospital	✓				✓	
Outreach programmes to prevent readmission of patients with COPD to hospital	✓		✓	✓	✓	
Ambulatory care at home for patients with chronic disease	✓		✓		✓	
Hospital admission risk programmes to prevent hospital admission of patients with chronic disease	✓					
Shared patient assessment and care planning	✓					
Self-management support	✓	✓	✓	✓	✓	✓
Chronic disease collaboratives	✓	✓		✓	✓	
Information and communication systems	✓	✓		✓	✓	✓

Source: Authors' own compilation.

Notes: CHF: Congestive heart failure; COPD: chronic obstructive pulmonary disease.

Fig. 8.2 *General practitioners' claims for chronic disease initiatives, July 2005 to October 2006*

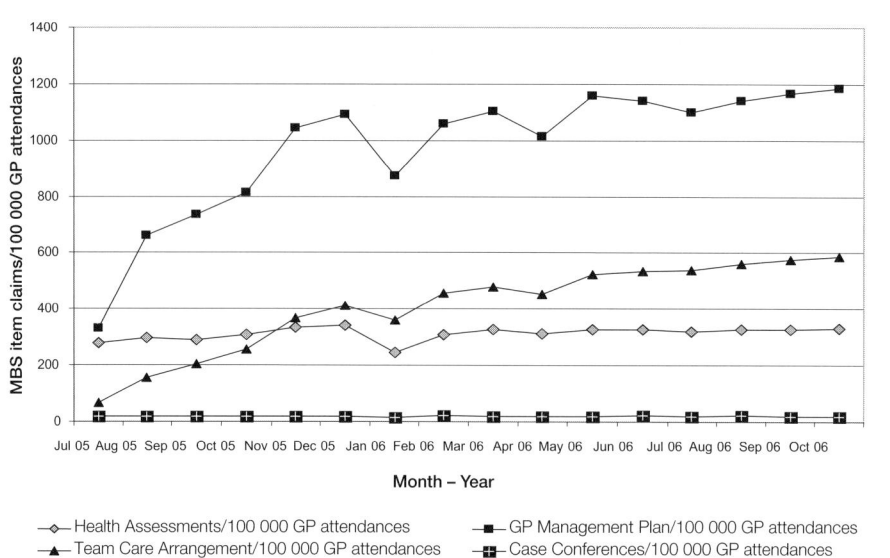

Source: Medicare online data (Australian Government Medicare Australia 2006b).

Notes: MBS: Medicare Benefits Schedule; GP: General practitioner.

by examining claims for health assessments, management plans, contingencies and TCAs (coordinated multidisciplinary care), as shown in Fig. 8.2. The figure illustrates that the more complicated initiatives, which involve liaison with other health professionals, are undertaken less frequently than, for example, health assessments.

Claims data for disease-specific incentives relating to diabetes, asthma and mental health provide another measure of uptake. For example, more than 90% of practices participating in the PIP have signed up for the PIP payments. However, the simultaneous advent of three different disease-focused programmes has proved challenging for general practice. Claims made for the SIPs have been variable across programmes, with lower uptake of the incentive related to asthma (Zwar et al. 2005). Other reasons for the variable uptake include the complexity of the programmes themselves, and factors related to the patients' views of the condition(s) (Fig. 8.3).

In contrast to other countries, such as the United States, private health insurers have so far had a limited role in chronic disease management, as they have been restricted to providing insurance for inpatient treatment provided in hospitals and for dental and allied health care. Despite this, some insurers have piloted chronic disease programmes for their members.

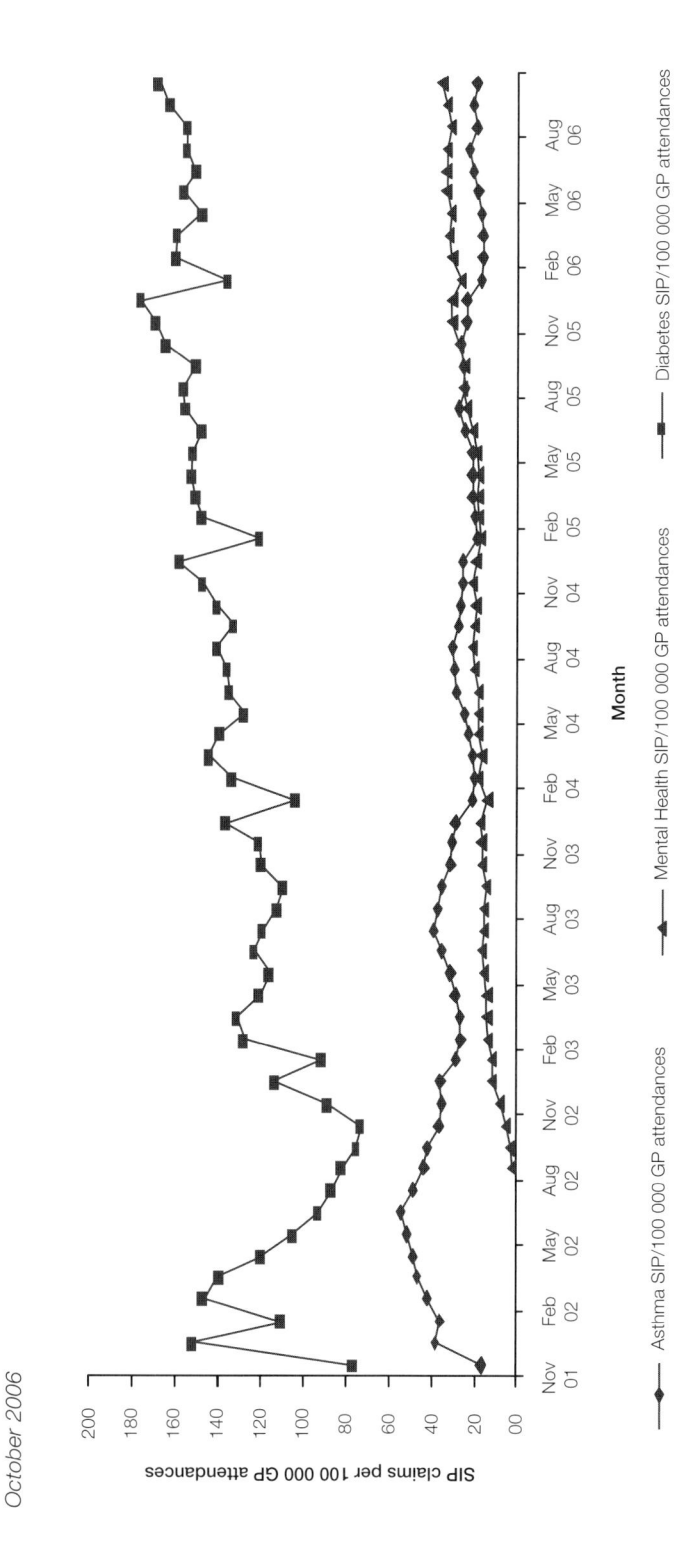

Fig. 8.3 Service Incentive Payment claims made by general practitioners in Australia for Asthma 3+, diabetes and mental health from November 2001 to October 2006

Source: Medicare online data (Australian Government Medicare Australia 2006b).

Notes: SIP: Service Incentive Payment; GP: General practitioner.

The level of population coverage by chronic disease programmes is difficult to estimate as most participants in programmes are not formally enrolled with a specific GP and an individual patient may be involved in multiple programmes or services. This is compounded in the Australian health system by the absence of patient registers in general practices.

Medicare Australia data for practices that participate in PIP provide an estimate of the population reach of the programmes adopted by those practices. For example, figures from August 2006 showed that the practices that had signed up to the asthma and diabetes PIPs had a coverage of 75% and 76% of the total population, respectively (Australian Government Medicare Australia 2006b).

In general terms, equity of access to chronic disease care in Australia is underpinned by the universal health insurance provided by Medicare. In 2004–2005, 75% of attendances in general practice were "bulk billed", with the provider invoicing the insurer directly (Australian Government Department of Health and Ageing 2005) and, as there is no payment by the patient for these consultations, chronic disease programmes provided by general practice are affordable. Exceptions occur in areas where GPs charge co-payments and patients have little choice but to pay them, as occurs in some rural and remote communities. Research looking specifically at equity of access to longer consultations has shown that, despite higher rates of chronic illness, patients living in poorer areas receive fewer extended general practice consultations than patients in more advantaged areas (Furler et al. 2002). There are particular barriers to access for Aboriginal and Torres Strait Islanders people, reflecting factors such as their poor socioeconomic status, cultural issues, service availability, and geographical remoteness. Despite efforts to increase access to services through Aboriginal Community Controlled Services, claims for PIP and other chronic disease items are substantially lower than for other Australians despite the higher burden of disease among the former.

The National Integrated Diabetes Programme

This section discusses the National Integrated Diabetes Programme (NIDP) as an illustrative example of a chronic disease care programme in Australia.

The incidence of type 2 diabetes in Australia is increasing, with over 7.4% of the population aged over 25 years having diabetes and a further 12.1% having impaired glucose tolerance (Dunstan et al. 2002). Direct annual health care costs of diabetes are estimated to be AUD 2.3 billion (€1.4 billion) per annum (McCarty et al. 1996).

Since the 1970s, Diabetes Centres have provided specialized multidisciplinary care. During the 1990s, they established shared care programmes with many

Divisions of General Practice (Burns et al. 2000). By 2004–2005, 114 of the 119 Divisions had specific programmes directed at diabetes, two thirds of which provided clinical services for patients with diabetes (Hordacre et al. 2006). A national diabetes supply scheme provides equipment and education in addition to the Pharmaceutical Benefits Scheme, which subsidizes medication. Nevertheless, up to 50% of patients attending general practice may receive sub-optimal care (Georgiou et al. 2004b).

In late 2001 the Commonwealth Government established the NIDP. This programme provides financial incentives for GPs, including a "sign on" payment if they establish a register for their patients with diabetes and a SIP in respect of each patient who completes an "annual cycle of care". The latter includes elements of regular assessment (blood pressure, BMI, HbA1c, lipids and the SNAP risk factors (smoking, nutrition, alcohol and physical activity)) and screening for complications (retinopathy, nephropathy, foot complications). There is an additional incentive for reaching a target level of patients completing the annual cycle. GPs are also able to claim for care plans on many of their patients with diabetes who require multidisciplinary care.

Diabetes self-management education is provided largely by specialist nurses and dieticians in Diabetes Centres, although the number of staff has been inadequate to meet the needs of all patients with diabetes.

A series of guidelines developed by the National Health and Medical Research Council (NHMRC) have been translated into guides for primary care. There has been limited electronic decision support for diabetes management in general practice, aside from a diabetes module which was incorporated into most of the common software packages used in general practice. Information systems remain somewhat fragmented, although better communication about diabetes between hospitals and general practice has been the focus of trials within the national e-health initiative. Between 1997 and 2003, many Divisions of General Practice established regional diabetes registers, based on a minimum clinical data set (Penn et al. 2004). These appear to have had a positive effect on the quality of care (Harris et al. 2002). However, few of these registers have been sustained in the long term.

An evaluation of the NIDP was conducted in 2005 but has not yet been made public. As mentioned previously, by 2006, over 90% of eligible practices had signed on for the diabetes PIP. Of these eligible practices, 70% had received SIPs and half of these practices had reached their target. An estimated 29% of patients with diabetes attending the "signed on" practices achieved the annual cycle of care, with levels being higher in disadvantaged than advantaged communities (Georgiou, Burns & Harris 2004a). In a cohort of patients on diabetes registers between 2000 and 2002, indicators of quality of care had improved and the mean levels of HbA1c, systolic blood pressure, diastolic blood pressure, low density lipoproteins, triglycerides and total cholesterol fell following the introduction of the NIDP (Georgiou et al. 2006).

A patient journey: Australia

In Australia, people with chronic diseases are typically diagnosed initially in one of three ways.

- They present to a GP and are screened (because of age or risk) for chronic diseases such as diabetes, hypertension or hyperlipidaemia.

- They present to a GP concerned about particular symptoms and as a result of this presentation a particular chronic disease is identified. For example, a person with undiagnosed diabetes and COPD may present to the GP because of increasing coughing, and in the course of the consultation that follows have both conditions identified.

- They experience an acute complication arising from a chronic disease and thus present to a GP or Emergency Department for treatment. The underlying chronic disease is then identified. For example, diabetes may be diagnosed following presentation to the Emergency Department with severe cellulitis.

Ongoing management of chronic disease is usually conducted in the general practice setting, as outlined earlier, supported intermittently by specialist services. Programmes have been implemented that assist people to move through the system, with an increased focus on prevention and self-management. Some initiatives focus on greater access to knowledge about medical conditions, including chronic conditions and associated risk factors. Underpinning these are notions that a more informed public will be empowered to self-manage on the one hand, and make more discriminating choices regarding appropriate service use on the other. An example of this approach is the Internet-based government initiative "HealthInsite" that provides quality information on a range of health topics (HealthInsite 2006). Call centres extend this concept. Health First in the Australian Capital Territory (ACT) provides a comprehensive web site on health and related services, easy access to health information, and telephone contact with registered nurses 24 hours a day, seven days a week (Health First 2006). The COAG is establishing a National Health Call Centre Network to provide reliable health care advice to people living in all parts of Australia.

Specific chronic disease management programmes have a limited role in Australia. There are some examples, typically sponsored by pharmaceutical companies in association with particular products. Data on the extent to which these are taken up are not publicly available. Several hospitals in New South Wales have recently adopted the Community Acute/Post Acute Care model that seeks to improve patient flows by offering inpatient hospital care to people in their homes (Australian Resource Centre for Healthcare Innovations 2006). However, communication between hospital and community providers is still not at optimal levels.

Health system features supporting programmes

Targets, standards and guidelines

The National Quality and Performance System (NQPS) for the Divisions of General Practice network was implemented by the Commonwealth Government in 2005, as a result of the 2003 evaluation of the role of the Divisions (Australian Government Department of Health and Ageing 2006d). It aims *"to drive continuous improvement across the Divisions network while allowing flexibility, support and recognition of the individual nature of Divisions"*. The NQPS includes performance indicators which assess a Division's achievements in five national priority areas: governance, prevention and early intervention, access, supporting integration and multidisciplinary care, and better management of chronic disease. In addition, regional priorities can be addressed through optional additional indicators. Indicators were developed at four different system levels: organizational, practice, community/family, and patient. A points system supports the indicators, with the intention that funding to the Divisions would ultimately be related to achievement of agreed targets. It was expected that, over time, indicators would be refined, or dropped, within existing priority areas, and new priority areas specified. The first round of reporting within this system occurred in 2006. NPQS data for 2005–2006 are available from the Australian Government Department of Health and Ageing (Australian Government Department of Health and Ageing 2008).

The data relevant to chronic disease only relate to continuing professional development activities undertaken by Divisions and are reported at State/Territory level. The NQPS does not link to a specific chronic disease programme per se, although both diabetes and asthma are included in the "Better Manage Chronic Disease" priority area mentioned earlier.

Implementation of performance assessment systems such as the NQPS has led to considerable debate, both within the medical profession and between providers and funders. There is concern as to the potential for risk being passed from the Government to providers or the difficulties faced by Divisions in being able to influence a particular doctor's behaviour. On the other hand, objective measures of performance may be seen as an opportunity to provide useful feedback to service providers and incentives to improve services. In addition, they have also been interpreted as potentially conveying evidence of value for money to the Government and wider community.

Health care workforce and capacity

New roles in chronic disease management have been slow to develop in Australian general practice, although the number of general practices with one or more nurses has increased from 23% in 2003 to 57% in 2005 (Australian Divisions of General Practice 2006). Support for GPs in rural areas to employ practice nurses (PIP practice nurse payment) was introduced as part of the 2001 Federal Budget; this was extended to urban areas facing workforce shortages. Practice nurses have become increasingly involved in conducting health assessments, as well as contributing to GPMPs and to TCAs.

Medicare item numbers were introduced in 2007 that would provide a rebate for the involvement of practice nurses in chronic disease care. Nurse practitioner positions exist, predominately in New South Wales, but almost all are in secondary or tertiary services, or in rural and remote settings. New roles have also developed at the hospital–community interface, such as specialist liaison nurses in NSW as part of the chronic care programme. In addition, pharmacists have been involved in pilots of screening programmes, self-management support, and medication reviews involving the elderly. The More Allied Health Services (MAHS) programme has provided funding for rural Divisions to employ allied health staff; 7% of whom were diabetes nurse specialists, 7% dieticians and 4% podiatrists (Hordacre et al. 2006). Aboriginal health workers are an important part of the primary health care workforce, predominately based in the network of Aboriginal Medical Services located both in rural and metropolitan areas. However, the Aboriginal Medical Services face continuing labour shortages.

Two recent reports have highlighted the challenge to Australia's health system presented by health workforce shortages. Both clearly identify chronic disease as a key driver for policies aimed at orientating the workforce towards future demands. The Productivity Commission Research Report *Australia's Health Workforce* (Productivity Commission 2005) and the Australian Medical Workforce Advisory Committee (AMWAC) report *The General Practice Workforce in Australia: supply and requirements to 2013* (AMWAC 2005) suggest a number of supply- and demand-side strategies aimed at addressing the workforce shortage. The Productivity Commission identified four broad strategies to overcome current shortages and uneven distribution of the health workforce:

- reducing underlying demand for health care through "wellness" and preventive strategies;

- short-term increases in education and training places in some areas and adequate clinical training capacity;
- greater emphasis on retention and re-entry; and
- improving the productivity and effectiveness of the available workforce, and its responsiveness to changing needs and pressures, without compromising safety and quality (Productivity Commission 2005).

The AMWAC has drawn attention to the current and estimated future shortage of GPs, with estimates of the shortfall ranging from 800 to 1300 GPs in 2002. Furthermore, it is estimated that there will be an annual shortage of entrants into the general practice workforce of approximately 400 to 500 Australian and overseas trained doctors between 2007 and 2013 (AMWAC 2005). Significant shortages of nurses are already projected to worsen over the next decade as many within the current cohort reach retirement age.

The Australian Government is responding to these problems with policies such as an expansion of medical student training, both in existing medical schools and by opening new schools, with the intention that the number of new medical graduates will expand by more than 60% over the next six years from the time of writing.

Examples of education and training initiatives specifically related to chronic disease exist across the continuum of health professional education and development. A focus on chronic diseases is evident and sometimes explicit in the undergraduate curricula in medical, nursing, pharmacy and allied health schools. For example, the Australian Medical Council, which accredits medical school programmes, includes standards that relate to chronic disease (Australian Medical Council Incorporated 2006) and the Royal Australian College of General Practitioners has a specific chapter in its general practice curriculum on chronic disease (RACGP 2006). There is an increasing array of courses designed to equip nurses for new or expanded roles in chronic disease management, including roles such as asthma educator and diabetes nurse educator. The Australian Practice Nursing Association (APNA) web site identifies 28 programmes (APNA 2007) and almost half of postgraduate courses are offered online only, with some having a mixture of online delivery and few face-to-face interactions.

Although interdisciplinary approaches to learning are generally uncommon, some continuing professional development programmes on chronic diseases have included a multidisciplinary component. For example, the "A Teams" from the National Asthma Council included asthma educators, GPs and respiratory physicians in the teams that delivered a structured asthma educational programme to GP and practice nurse audiences (National Asthma Council Australia 2006).

Regulation of health professional practice is largely undertaken within State and Territory jurisdictions. The processes are generic rather than specifically focused on chronic disease, although extended roles for professionals would require appropriate recognition by the relevant board. Once registration is obtained in one Australian State or Territory, application (on payment of a fee) can be made to other jurisdictions to have the registration recognized. In each State and Territory jurisdiction there are formally constituted bodies to deal with complaints.

The aforementioned 2005 report *Australia's Health Workforce* by the Productivity Commission identifies some potentially wide-ranging changes to the system (Productivity Commission 2005). In education and training an intergovernmental agreement on clinical training places is proposed, as is an increased focus on multidisciplinary/interdisciplinary training. New kinds of health workers are envisaged, as are new roles for existing health professionals. Accreditation of health professionals is being consolidated under a new national regime, and funding and payment mechanisms are to be better aligned to achieve desired outcomes. Although a number of these issues have attracted considerable public discussion, full implementation would require radical reform to the system. This would be contrary to the historical precedent that has been set by the Australian Government, which has favoured incremental change in the health arena.

Evaluation and lessons learned

In principle, all programmes implemented by the Australian Government are formally evaluated within three to five years of their implementation. Most commonly, evaluations are outsourced to independent contractors through approved tendering processes. The evaluation questions are designed to explore the appropriateness of the programme, its effectiveness and efficiency in meeting its intended aims, and to provide insight into the value for money that the programme represents. The resulting evaluation reports are designed to inform the Australian Government in the first instance, and may or may not subsequently be made public. Decisions to continue, modify or discontinue programmes are informed by evaluations, but they are not necessarily determined by them (Box 8.3).

The coordinated care trials of the 1990s represented a major investment by the Australian Government in developing the evidence base for improved care coordination for people with chronic and complex illness. However, interventions did not lead to better outcomes in terms of quality of life, rates of hospitalization, readmission or length of stay (Esterman & Den-Tovim 2002). The Enhanced Primary Care package which followed has been evaluated in terms of uptake (Wilkinson et al. 2003, Blakeman et al. 2001), and demonstrated that GPs had difficulty in incorporating multidisciplinary care into routine practice due to the way Australian general practice is structured and remunerated. Barriers to uptake

> **Box 8.3 Evaluating the Australian Asthma 3+ Visit Plan**
>
> The Australian Asthma Management Plan was adapted into a series of planned visits for general practice care of asthma called the Asthma 3+ Visit Plan. It incorporated financial incentives for general practitioners (GPs); a Practice Incentives Program (PIP) sign-on payment and a Service Incentive Payment (SIP). For a GP to claim the Asthma 3+ Visit Plan SIP (SIP-asthma), a patient must have had at least three asthma-related consultations over a period between 4 weeks and 4 months. Consultations must have covered diagnosis and assessment of severity, review of asthma-related medication, provision of a written asthma action plan, and patient education. Plan implementation was evaluated at local and national levels by researchers independent of government, using multiple methods including eliciting views from GPs (surveys) and service users (interviews), analysis of Medicare data, and focus groups comprising both service users and providers, with an additional component seeking views from Aboriginal Community Controlled Health Services and Aboriginal and Torres Strait Islander people (Beilby et al. 2004, Zwar et al. 2005).
>
> The evaluations revealed several important issues, including difficulties in getting people with asthma to return for all three visits and the challenges that GPs were faced with when attempting to integrate the relatively inflexible structure of the plan into routine practice. Obstacles included practice workload, inability to administer the relatively complex payment system in the absence of sophisticated practice administration systems, along with time and staff shortages. Based on these findings, it was recommended to revise the general practice incentive to an annual cycle of care that comprises a minimum of two visits for all patients diagnosed with asthma. In response, the Government launched an Asthma Cycle of Care initiative (from 1 November 2006) reducing the number of visits to two and increasing the time permitted to complete the cycle to one year, while maintaining the content of the Asthma 3+ Visit Plan. Yet, despite these modifications, there has been little change in the uptake of this approach, indicating the significance of other barriers to changing practice.

included issues regarding time (or lack thereof), organization, communication, education and resources (Blakeman et al. 2001). Challenges related to care planning included lack of knowledge among other health care professionals and asymmetry of incentives, so creating disincentives for involvement of other health professionals (Blakeman, Zwar & Harris 2002). Case conferences proved even more difficult, with the logistics of organizing a case conference being perceived as an insurmountable barrier for most GPs and only a limited number have been undertaken (Harris 2002, Mitchell et al. 2002).

There has been little research to date on the impact of care plans on patient outcomes, with the exception of diabetes care. For example, following the introduction of the National Integrated Diabetes Programme, a cohort of patients on diabetes registers was monitored and showed improvements in intermediate outcomes (Georgiou et al. 2006). One other study found improved adherence to guidelines for diabetes care. Metabolic control and cardiovascular risk factors improved for patients who had multidisciplinary care implemented (Zwar et al. 2007). The study was, however, not able to establish whether the observed improvement was due to the care plan prompting a more comprehensive review of diabetes care, whether it was attributable to improved teamwork and coordination of care, or both.

The elements of the demonstration projects that focused on self-management within the Sharing Health Care Initiative have also been evaluated. Using observational studies, positive effects on improved health outcomes, better quality of life and reduced use of health services have been reported (Australian Government Department of Health and Ageing 2005). However, so far, self-management elements have not been well integrated with mainstream general practice (Zwar et al. 2006). The demonstration projects have not yet been linked with EPC plans and it is likely that the vast majority of GPs would be unaware of these projects or see how self-management could be incorporated into the care plans they are developing. Harris et al. (2002) compared the care provided by GPs that used a diabetes shared care register and those who did not, demonstrating that care provided by those who used a shared care register was more consistent with clinical practice guidelines, thus illustrating the potential impact of decision support and clinical information systems on care outcomes.

In general terms, there has been a clear trend towards increasing research on chronic disease in primary care in Australia, evidenced by the increase in publications since the early 2000s and by the increasing uptake of this research in chronic disease policy. The Australian Primary Health Care Research Institute has recently completed a series of systematic reviews targeting national policy priorities, including chronic disease, models of care, and the workforce (Australian Primary Healthcare Research Institute 2006). In addition to the production of the reports themselves, an explicit goal also exists to increase the capacity of researchers to address policy questions and of policy advisors to use research.

Investing in the future

Based on the National Chronic Disease Strategy and the 2006 commitments of the Council of Australian Governments to the Better Health for all Australians package, the following vision and policy direction for Australia in the short-to-medium term can be articulated:

- There will a continued focus on person-centred care and self-management. This will be supported by a range of initiatives including, for example, call centres, greater use of recall and reminder systems, and care planning. Although formal patient registration with a particular general practice is not likely to occur in the short term, the benefits – in terms of better outcomes – that result from patients with chronic diseases being affiliated with a "usual" general practice will be emphasized. Health inequalities will be identified and addressed.

- There will be a particular focus on the health needs of Aboriginal and Torres Strait Islanders, with innovations within existing health service models designed to improve all health outcomes, including chronic diseases.

- The health system will give greater emphasis to health promotion and disease prevention activities, both through population-level interventions and by making greater use of an increasingly integrated primary care sector. It will also continue to emphasize the importance of making use of the existing evidence base to inform chronic disease management, while at the same time prospectively collecting key data and conducting research to develop that evidence base. Research priorities will include factors that enhance effectiveness and efficiency while maintaining quality, and factors that promote sustainability.

- The nature of the health workforce will change, with roles for some workers being extended, allowing them to undertake new activities that support chronic disease management. New kinds of health workers will be deployed, including a variation on the "physician assistant", trained to support people with chronic disease in community settings. There will be an ongoing focus on prevention of avoidable hospitalizations and procedures and management of chronic disease within the community.

- New strategic partnerships will be established. These will include jurisdictional partnerships addressing, for example, innovative approaches to the pooling of funds, as well as partnerships between organizations and institutions within the private and public sectors. A variety of approaches to governance may be used to support these partnerships, with the objective of enhancing health outcomes for those with chronic diseases, where possible realizing efficiency gains.

- There will continue to be a focus on IT and related infrastructure. This will include greater use of recall and reminder systems, greater use of electronic health records, more electronic decision supports, and greater use of electronic health data moving across the health system to provide timely information for patients and health care providers. IT will increasingly be aligned to a national set of standards.

However, although this vision is reasonably well outlined in Australian government documents, the strategies and goals required to realize it are set out at a very general level only. There remains a substantial amount of work to be done to develop strategies, goals and markers for success at regional or institutional/organizational levels. It is a strength to have a nationally agreed vision related to chronic disease. Yet it is a potential threat for that vision's realization to be dependent on a large amount of local activity from disparate entities. The Commonwealth Government together with the State and Territory governments have made a substantial financial commitment to realizing improved chronic disease and mental health outcomes.

Table 8.2 presents an analysis of some key factors pertinent to achieving this vision, including some human, intellectual, financial and social capital considerations. Not only are these relevant to initial implementation, but they are also important in terms of sustaining any reforms. The reforms planned are incremental rather than radical, and the fundamental division of responsibilities in health care between the Commonwealth Government and State governments looks likely to remain. The jury is still out on whether these reforms will be able to be carried through and whether they will be sufficient to respond to the challenges of the chronic disease burden.

Conclusion

Australia has a complex health system with a number of features that impact directly on attempts to give a greater priority to chronic disease. These features include split responsibilities for different parts of the system between State or Territory and governments and the Commonwealth Government, strong traditions of professional independence, and the structural orientation of Medicare towards acute and episodic care through fee-for-service payments.

Chronic disease places very substantial demands on the Australian health system, and projections point to this demand increasing. There have been a number of responses aimed at improving chronic disease management. At the federal level these have largely focused on general practice with the introduction of some incentive payments for chronic disease management, together with new Medicare items aimed at increasing multidisciplinary care and care provided by practice nurses. In comparison with other countries, primary health care organizations have relatively underdeveloped service delivery and development roles, with most of their efforts focused on quality improvement and practice support. An additional complication is the current workforce shortage, affecting GPs and nurses in particular. These issues are expected to remain problematic over the next decade, notwithstanding a number of policy initiatives aimed at addressing the shortages.

At the same time, there are encouraging signs that, within this complex system, it is possible to realize improvements, such as those in diabetes care and in the use of the EPC package. Policy initiatives also take account of evidence, as illustrated by the modifications to the asthma care cycle.

The COAG has made very substantial funding commitments in areas related to chronic disease management over the next five years from the time of writing. The challenge in Australia is to formulate and implement specific innovative service delivery models for patients that are less fragmented, draw together the efforts of all levels of government, and are sustainable given both the projected workforce and consumer demand.

Table 8.2 Chronic disease management in Australia: strengths and weaknesses

	Strengths	Weaknesses	Opportunities	Threats
Policy content	NCDS consistent with current models for chronic disease management including focus on self-care and care in the community	Fee-for-service payments, medically orientated MBS, designed for acute and episodic health care needs rather than chronic disease care	Innovative approaches broadening range of services funded through MBS to include chronic disease prevention activities and support for other providers Greater focus on prevention through ABHI Greater use of evidence in chronic disease management More self-management	System has little if any surplus capacity beyond responding to acute and episodic demand to redirect health services into chronic disease care
Policy consistency	NCDS provides agreed cross-jurisdictional framework COAG commitment to Better Health for All Australians package COAG has established an implementation group for the package	Implementation dependent on state/territory/regional/local responses Funding of health services is divided between federal and state/territory jurisdictions	Blueprint for nationwide surveillance of chronic diseases and associated determinants has potential to provide information to inform NCDS policy development	Momentum for common national approach is lost Federal/state divide introduces divergent policies in response to local pressures
Short- versus long-term perspective	COAG commitment to Better Health for All Australians package commits funds for 5 years from 2006	Plans for expenditure of committed funds still under development	Substantial funds available to implement enhanced prevention and care services for chronic disease	Planning consumes implementation time Resulting from lag in actually spending announced funds, other spending priorities including from other sectors could emerge

(cont.)

Table 8.2 *(cont.)*

	Strengths	Weaknesses	Opportunities	Threats
Influence of electoral cycles	Broad directions of NCDS likely to be acceptable to all political factions at both federal and state/territory levels	Lobbyists promote particular chronic diseases	Greater awareness of chronic disease issues	Greater demand for services from an already stressed health system
Impact of institutional framework	Highly variable depending on jurisdiction and level of the system in which the institution operates	Resourcing issues likely to arise with institutional claims for more resources	Innovative approaches to governance and collaboration across institutions at local and regional levels lead to enhanced services	Institutions refuse to "buy in" Private and public sectors do not invest in necessary infrastructure
Impact of macro-economic conditions/ constraints	Use of large public sector budget surpluses to improve health outcomes Substantial COAG commitment over next 5 years Despite shortages, a generally well-trained and motivated workforce	Increased pressure to achieve efficiencies/reduce costs Lack of alignment of fee-for-service funding mechanisms with best practice chronic disease management	Trials of commissioning/funds pooling/other models to optimize local/regional services	Resistance to any change from established providers Workforce shortages Inflexibility in current training arrangements Economic downturn reduces available funds

Source: Authors' own compilation.

Note: NCDS: National Chronic Disease Strategy; MBS: Medicare Benefits Schedule; ABHI: Australian Better Health Initiative; COAG: Council of Australian Governments.

References

ABS (2005). *The health and welfare of Australia's Aboriginal and Torres Strait Islander Peoples, 2005*. Canberra, Australian Bureau of Statistics.

ABS (2007) [web site]. Canberra, Australian Bureau of Statistics (http://www.abs.gov.au/websitedbs/d3310114.nsf/Home/Home?OpenDocument, accessed 4 January 2007).

Australian Divisions of General Practice (2006). *National practice nurse workforce survey report*. Manuka, Australian Divisions of General Practice.

Australian Government Department of Health and Ageing (2005). *National evaluation of the Sharing Health Care Initiative. Final technical report*. Canberra, Australian Government Department of Health and Ageing.

Australian Government Department of Health and Ageing (2006a) [web site]. Rural health services. Canberra, Australian Government Department of Health and Ageing (http://www.health.gov.au/internet/wcms/publishing.nsf/Content/ruralhealth-services-index.htm, accessed 28 April 2006).

Australian Government Department of Health and Ageing (2006b) [web site]. Health Connect: Northern Territory. Canberra, Australian Government Department of Health and Ageing (http://www.health.gov.au/internet/hconnect/publishing.nsf/Content/nt-1lp, accessed 4 January 2007).

Australian Government Department of Health and Ageing (2006c) [web site]. Healthy for life. Canberra, Australian Government Department of Health and Ageing (http://www.health.gov.au/healthyforlife, accessed March 2007).

Australian Government Department of Health and Ageing (2006d) [web site]. Divisions of General Practice Programme – Programme Guidelines for use by the Divisions Network. Canberra, Australian Government Department of Health and Ageing (http://www.health.gov.au/internet/wcms/publishing.nsf/Content/health-pcd-prog-divisions-guidelines, accessed 5 January 2007).

Australian Government Department of Health and Ageing (2007a) [web site]. Health priorities. Canberra, Australian Government Department of Health and Ageing (http://www.health.gov.au/internet/wcms/publishing.nsf/Content/Health+Priorities-1, accessed 4 January 2007).

Australian Government Department of Health and Ageing (2007b). *Medicare health checks for Aboriginal and Torres Strait Islander Australians. Fact sheet*. Canberra, Australian Government Department of Health and Ageing.

Australian Government Department of Health and Ageing (2008) [web site]. National Quality and Performance System. Canberra, Australian Government Department of Health and Ageing (http://www.healthconnect.gov.au/internet/main/publishing.nsf/Content/health-pcd-programs-divisions-NQPS, accessed May 2008).

Australian Government Medicare Australia (2006a) [web site]. About Medicare Australia. Greenway, Australian Government Medicare Australia (http://www.medicareaustralia.gov.au/about/index.shtml, accessed 22 December 2006).

Australian Government Medicare Australia (2006b) [web site]. Medicare health statistics. Greenway, Australian Government Medicare Australia (http://www.medicareaustralia.gov.au/providers/health_statistics/statistical_reporting/medicare.htm, accessed 30 November 2006).

Australian Government Medicare Australia (2008) [web site]. Incentives & allowances. Greenway, Australian Governmenr Medicare Australia (http://www.medicareaustralia.gov.au/provider/incentives/index.shtml, accessed 13 August 2008).

Australian Indigenous HealthInfoNet (2007) [web site] MT Lawley, WA, Australian Indigenous HealthInfoNet (http://www.healthinfonet.ecu.edu.au/, accessed March 2007).

AIHW (2006) [web site]. Australia's national agency for health and welfare statistics and information. Canberra, Australian Institute of Health and Welfare (http://www.aihw.gov.au/index.cfm, accessed 22 December 2006).

AIHW (2001). *Expenditures on health services for Aboriginal and Torres Strait Islander people 1998–1999*. Canberra, Australian Institute of Health and Welfare and Commonwealth, Department of Health and Aged Care.

Australian Medical Council Incorporated (2006). *Part 2 of the Australian Medical Council's guidelines; assessment and accreditation of medical schools: standards and procedures 2002*. Canberra, Australian Medical Council Incorporated.

AMWAC (2005). *The general practice workforce in Australia: supply and requirements to 2013*. Sydney, Australian Medical Workforce Advisory Committee.

APNA (2007) [web site]. Education, training, career development. Melbourne, Australian Practice Nurses Association (http://www.apna.asn.au/displaycommon.cfm?an=5, accessed 5 January 2007).

APCC (2006) [web site]. National Primary Care Collaboratives. Adelaide, Australian Primary Care Collaboratives (http://www.apcc.org.au/, accessed 13 August 2008).

Australian Primary Healthcare Research Institute (2006) [web site]. ANU College of Medicine and Health Sciences. Stream Four. Canberra, Australian Primary Healthcare Research Institute (http://www.anu.edu.au/aphcri/Spokes_Research_Program/Stream_Four.php, accessed 5 January 2007).

Australian Resource Centre for Healthcare Innovations (2006) [web site]. Community acute/post acute care (CAPAC). Wallsend, NSW, Australian Resource Centre for Healthcare Innovations (http://www.archi.net.au/e-library/build/moc/capac, accessed 5 January 2007).

Bailie R et al. (2007). Indigenous health: The potential and requirements of continuous quality improvement for effective and sustainable services. *Medical Journal of Australia*, 186:525–527.

Beilby J et al. (2004). *Evaluation of the Asthma 3+ Visit Plan*. Adelaide, University of Adelaide and University of New South Wales.

Blakeman T et al. (2001). Evaluating general practitioners' views about the implementation of the Enhanced Primary Care Medicare items. *Medical Journal of Australia*, 175:95–98.

Blakeman T, Zwar N, Harris M (2002). Evaluating general practitioners' views on the enhanced primary care items for care planning and case conferencing: a one year follow-up. *Australian Family Physician*, 31:582–585.

Britt H et al. (2002). *General practice activity in Australia: 2001–2002*. Canberra, Australian Institute of Health and Welfare.

Burns J et al. (2000). *National Divisions Diabetes Programme Data Collation Project. Volume 2: Divisions of General Practice – Diabetes profiles. Division and programme descriptions.* Sydney, Centre for General Practice Integration Studies, School of Community Medicine, University of New South Wales.

COAG (2006a). *Better health for all Australians. Action plan*. Canberra, Council of Australian Governments.

COAG (2006b). *National action plan on mental health 2006–2011*. Canberra, Council of Australian Governments.

Dunstan D et al. (2002). The rising prevalence of diabetes and impaired glucose tolerance: the Australian Diabetes, Obesity and Lifestyle Study. *Diabetes Care*, 25:829–834.

Esterman A & Den-Tovim D (2002). The Australian coordinated care trials: success or failure? *Medical Journal of Australia*, 177:469–470.

Farmer L, Knight A, Ford D (2005). Systems change in Australian general practice: early impact of the National Primary Care Collaboratives. *Australian Family Physician*, 34:44–46.

Furler J et al. (2002). The inverse care law revisited: impact of disadvantaged location on accessing longer GP consultation times. *Medical Journal of Australia*, 177:80-83.

Georgiou A et al. (2006). Monitoring change in diabetes care using diabetes registers: experience from Divisions of General Practice. *Australian Family Physician*, 35:77–80.

Georgiou A, Burns J, Harris M (2004a). GP Claims for completing diabetes "cycle of care". *Australian Family Physician*, 33:755–757.

Georgiou A et al. (2004b). *Divisions Diabetes & CVD Quality Improvement Project. Analysis of Division-based diabetes register data (2000–2002)*. Sydney, Centre for General Practice Integration Studies, University of New South Wales.

Harris M (2002). Case conferences in general practice: time for a rethink? *Medical Journal of Australia*, 177:93–94.

Harris M et al. (2002). Quality of care provided by general practitioners using or not using division-based registers. *Medical Journal of Australia*, 177:250–252.

Health First (2006) [web site]. Canberra, Health First (http://www.healthfirst.net.au/providersearch.ser, accessed 5 January 2007)

HealthInsite (2006) [web site]. About Healthinsite. Canberra, HealthInsite (http://www.healthinsite.gov.au/static/About_HealthInsite, accessed 5 January 2007).

Hordacre A et al. (2006). *Making the connections. Report of the 2004–2005 Annual Survey of Divisions of General Practice*. Adelaide, Primary Health Care Research and Information Service, Department of General Practice, Flinders University, and Australian Government Department of Health and Ageing.

Jordan J, Osbourne R (2007). Chronic disease self-management programs: challenges ahead. *Medicare Journal of Australia*, 186:84–87.

Mayers N, Couzos S (2004). Towards health equity through an adult health check for Aboriginal and Torres Strait Islander people. *Medical Journal of Australia*, 181:531–532.

McCarty D et al. (1996). *The rise and rise of diabetes in Australia, 1996. A review of statistics, trends and costs*. Canberra, Diabetes Australia.

Mitchell G et al. (2002). General practitioners' attitudes to case conferences: how can we increase participation? *Medical Journal of Australia*, 177:95–97.

National Asthma Council Australia (2002). *Asthma management handbook*. Melbourne, National Asthma Council Australia.

National Asthma Council Australia (2006) [web site]. Newsletter 2005. Melbourne, National Asthma Council Australia (http://www.nationalasthma.org.au/html/newsletter/2005/index.asp, accessed 5 January 2007).

National Health Priority Action Council (2005). *National chronic disease strategy*. Canberra, Australian Government Department of Health and Ageing.

NSW Government Treasury (2007) [web site]. NSW Treasury 2006–07 budget papers. Sydney, NSW Government Treasury (http://www.treasury.nsw.gov.au/bp06-07/bpapers, accessed 13 August 2008).

Penn D et al. (2004). Evolution of a register recall system to enable the delivery of better quality of care in general practice. *Health Informatics Journal*, 10:163–174.

Productivity Commission (2005). *Australia's health workforce*. Productivity Commission research report. Canberra, Productivity Commission.

RACGP (2006) [web site]. Education and Training. Canberra, Royal Australian College of General Practitioners (http://www.racgp.org.au/curriculum, accessed 5 January 2007).

RACGP (2000). *Standards and guidelines for the Enhanced Primary Care Medicare Benefits Schedule items*. Canberra, Royal Australian College of General Practitioners, Commonwealth Department of Health and Ageing.

Scott M (2002). The NSW Aboriginal vascular health program. *NSW Public Health Bulletin*, 13:152–154.

Si D et al. (2005). Assessing health centre systems for guiding improvement in diabetes care. *BioMed Central Health Services Research*, 5:56.

State Government of Victoria Department of Human Services (2006) [web site]. Primary care partnerships. Victoria, State Government of Victoria Department of Human Services (http://www.health.vic.gov.au/pcps/, accessed 4 January 2007).

Vagholkar S et al. (2007). Multidisciplinary care plans for patients with diabetes: what do they contain? *Australian Family Physician*, 36:279–282.

Wagner E, Austin B, Von Korff M (1996). Organizing care for patients with chronic illness. *Milbank Quarterly*, 74:511–544.

Wilkinson D et al. (2003). *Evaluation of the enhanced primary care Medicare Benefits Schedule (MBS) items and the general practice education, support and community linkages programme*. Canberra, Commonwealth Department of Health and Ageing (Final Report July 2003).

Williams et al. (2007). Sustaining chronic disease management in primary care: lessons from a demonstration project. *Australian Journal of Primary Health*, 13:121–128.

Woolcock et al. (1989). Asthma management plan. *Medical Journal of Australia*, 151:650–653.

WHO (1981). *WHO's global strategy for health for all by the year 2000*. Geneva, World Health Organization.

Zwar N et al. (2005). General practitioner views on barriers and facilitators to implementation of the Asthma 3+ Visit Plan. *Medical Journal of Australia*, 183:64–67.

Zwar N et al. (2006). *Systematic review of chronic disease management*. Sydney, Research Centre for Primary Health Care and Equity, School of Public Health and Community Medicine, University of New South Wales.

Zwar N et al. (2007). Do multidisciplinary care plans result in better care for patients with type 2 diabetes? *Australian Family Physician*, 36:85–89.

Chapter 9
Canada

Izzat Jiwani, Carl-Ardy Dubois

Context

Canadian health care has to be understood within the historical context of Canadian fiscal and social policy and the constitutional division of power between the federal and provincial governments. The British North America Act of 1867 had given control of the organization and delivery of health care services to the 13 provinces and territories, while leaving most of the taxation powers with the federal Government. Provincial governments receive funding for health, education and social services through a transfer funding mechanism, which evolved from the original cost-sharing arrangements supporting Medicare. The evolution of health care in Canada has resulted in a predominantly publicly financed health care system, but delivered through private for profit-making and non-profit-making organizations. The enduring effect of these historical arrangements, coupled with the contemporary interests of key stakeholders and socioeconomic and political contexts, continue to impact on health policy.

The federal Government is responsible for protecting the health and security of Canadians by setting standards for the national Medicare system, and for ensuring that the provinces follow the principles of public health care enshrined in the 1984 Canada Health Act. It also has key responsibilities in the public health domain, drug and food safety regulation, data collection and health research (Marchildon 2005). Additionally, it has direct jurisdiction over health services for the armed forces and the Royal Canadian Mounted Police, First Nations and Inuit people who are not covered under provincial and territory health insurance schemes, along with veterans and inmates of federal penitentiaries. Hospital services and physicians' public health care services are insured under the Canada Health Act and funded by provincial governments. Most hospitals in Canada are private non-profit-making organizations, and physicians practise privately with a fee-for-service payment mechanism in place. Provincial governments negotiate remuneration for physicians' services with provincial medical associations. The federal Government can withhold a portion of the transfer of funds to a province should health providers impose user fees or extra billing for "medically necessary services". This effectively blocks the provision of private treatment for any care that is available publicly.

The nature of the Canadian Federation means that provinces differ in their coverage of most of the medical services that are outside of the package of publicly funded services, as well as in the organization of health care. The provincial governments are responsible for coverage of prescription pharmaceuticals, providing an array of public services, and funding or subsidizing, directly or indirectly, some long-term care and home care services. Most provinces only cover prescription pharmaceuticals for select groups such as seniors and those on social assistance; the rest of the population obtains pharmaceutical coverage through private and employer-sponsored insurance, or through out-of-pocket payments. In most provinces, health services at provincial level are organized, primarily, by Regional Health Authorities (RHAs), which coordinate and deliver services to a defined geographic population (Church & Barker 1998, Denis 2002). RHAs were implemented in the 1990s with the overarching goals of achieving financial, clinical, organizational and epidemiological targets, but they vary in their functions and format across the country. Ontario, which had not thus far decentralized health care, has also started implementing a form of regionalization, the local health integration networks (LHINs).

Analysing the response

Approaches to chronic disease management

In response to an ageing population and the growing burden of chronic disease, the federal and the provincial governments have developed policies and initiatives that target both promotion of healthy lifestyles and prevention of chronic diseases.

National response

In September 2002 the Federal, Provincial and Territorial Ministers of Health announced the Integrated Pan-Canadian Healthy Living Strategy, a scheme that was subsequently approved in 2005. This strategy has the goal of promoting healthy living, which is defined as practices that are consistent with improving or maintaining health (including both individual and environmental factors) (Secretariat for the Intersectoral Healthy Living Network, Living Task Group & Advisory Committee on Population Health and Health Security 2005). The strategy envisages an integrated approach, focusing on multiple settings for health, and encouraging the use of best practices. Other initiatives at both federal and provincial levels have focused on prevention of chronic diseases and are implemented in various settings, including schools, communities, and worksites, with a clear focus on established lifestyle-related factors, such as physical activity, healthy eating and tobacco use.

The national initiatives include:

- the **Canadian Diabetes Strategy** that seeks to prevent diabetes where feasible, and help Canadians better manage the disease and its complications;

- the **Canadian Heart Health Initiative,** which supports programmes that aim to demonstrate the efficacy of evidence-based public health approaches to preventing and reducing cardiovascular disease and to build capacity in the public health system for planning and implementing effective provincial and community heart health interventions;

- the **Federal Tobacco Control Strategy** whose activities build on a framework with four mutually reinforcing components: protection, prevention, cessation and harm reduction, supplemented by effective use of public education campaigns to reach all Canadians;

- the **Office of Nutrition Policy and Promotion (Health Canada)**, which promotes the nutritional health and well-being of Canadians by defining, promoting and implementing evidence-based nutrition policies, and providing guidance for the population as a whole, such as Canada's Food Guide to Healthy Eating.

The Centre for Chronic Disease Prevention and Control (CCDPC), established in 2004 and operating under the Public Health Agency of Canada has implemented a Best Practices Portal for Health Promotion and Chronic Disease Prevention (CCDPC 2007), and a disease surveillance web site. It compiles the most up-to-date statistics on major chronic diseases in Canada, and includes trends in mortality by province and territory. The web site also provides cancer data and a National Diabetes Surveillance System (NDSS).

There are other key strategies implemented by the federal Government that have directly or indirectly assisted the provinces to develop responses to chronic disease. For example, the Primary Health Care Transition Fund has, over a 6-year period (2000–2006), supported the provinces in improving primary care by establishing multidisciplinary teams. In addition, Canada's four western

> **Box 9.1 The Western Health Information Collaborative**
>
> The Western Health Information Collaborative (WHIC) is a partnership of the provinces of British Columbia, Saskatchewan, Alberta and Manitoba and funded through Health Canada's Primary Health Care Transition Fund (WHIC 2006). It has focused on developing data and message exchange standards to enable health care providers to access data in an integrated and easily accessible form and thereby support chronic disease management. It enhanced British Columbia's chronic disease management Toolkit so that it supports the WHIC chronic disease management data standards in each of the participating provinces.

provinces (British Columbia, Saskatchewan, Alberta and Manitoba) received CAD 8 million (€5.4 million) in federal funding for a chronic disease management "Infoway" (the Western Health Information Collaborative, WHIC) (see Box 9.1) to implement common data standards and electronic messages related to three chronic diseases: diabetes, hypertension and renal failure.

Provincial policies and initiatives

Most provinces and territories in Canada have identified chronic disease as one of their key priorities and each province has developed specific strategies in response. Most provinces have their own specific frameworks for healthy living and the prevention of chronic disease. These include the British Columbia Health Living Targets for 2010 (2005), the Alberta Healthy Living Network (2003), and the Nova Scotia Chronic Disease Prevention Strategy (Dalhousie University 2003). Currently one of the most detailed and specific plans for tackling chronic disease is Ontario's Cancer 2020 Plan (Canadian Cancer Society and CCO 2003). This strategy encompasses multiple determinants of cancer: tobacco use, diet and nutrition, healthy body weight, physical activity, alcohol consumption, occupational and environmental carcinogens, radiation exposure, viral infections, and screening services.

The following section briefly describes selected provincial strategies for chronic disease management.

The Government of **British Columbia**, in collaboration with a range of stakeholders, has launched a province-wide chronic disease management programme, using an "Expanded Chronic Care Model", which incorporates health promotion and disease prevention (Government of British Columbia Ministry of Health 2007). As part of this programme, report cards are published regularly on disease prevalence, incidence, patient survival, costs, and performance gaps, using information from newly established chronic disease registries. A web site has been created to give patients and practitioners access to information and tools to support them in managing chronic diseases. Other initiatives include: the ActNow BC strategy that requires each government department to develop strategies and actions that will reduce the prevalence of common risk factors contributing to chronic disease; structured chronic disease management collaboratives to support integration of best practices in chronic care into clinical practice; a financial incentive programme, including a Full Service Family Practice Incentive Program to support evidence-based management of congestive heart failure, diabetes and hypertension; patient registries for selected diseases; professional development activities designed to enhance skills in self-evaluation, patient self-management coaching, and use of web-based and personal digital assistant (PDA) technology in clinical practice; and self-management training and support for patients.

In 2005 the Health Quality Council in **Saskatchewan** launched the Saskatchewan Chronic Disease Management Collaborative as a major initiative to improve the care and health of people living with coronary artery disease and diabetes, and to improve access to physicians (Health Quality Council 2005). Running in two waves, with the second wave launched in 2006 and due to end in 2009, the Collaborative brings together all 13 health regions in Saskatchewan, family physician practices, First Nations organizations, and community health care providers, among others. Guided by the evidence-based principles of good chronic care (Expanded Chronic Care Model), health care professionals and organizations become part of a network of experts and fellow learners (the Collaborative Learning Model) in order to gain skills in performing changes that make sense in each unique setting (Model for Improvement).

Early findings from the Collaborative indicate considerable improvements in the quality care of those with chronic disease (Health Council of Canada 2007), with practices involved reporting, for example, a 39% improvement in screening for kidney disease, a 26% improvement in appropriate prescribing of anti-platelet medication for patients with diabetes to reduce the risk of heart attacks and strokes, a 6% improvement in the proportion of patients with diabetes whose HbA1c was 7% or less (as recommended by expert guidelines), and a 4% improvement in the proportion of patients with coronary artery disease whose blood pressure was controlled.

Alberta has established a province-wide electronic health record system, the Alberta NetCare Electronic Health Record. Alberta's two regional health authorities, Capital Health in Edmonton and the Calgary Health Region, provide examples of some of the best practices in Canada. Thus, the Chronic Disease Management Programme in Capital Health includes regionalized programmes with centralized referrals; a regional electronic medical/health records system; a triage process to ensure patients obtain the right service from the right provider at the right time; standardized pathways for assessment,

> **Box 9.2 Community care coordinators in Calgary Health Region**
>
> As part of Calgary Health Region's chronic disease management strategy, community care coordinators (nurses) carry out case management. A registered nurse case manager sees patients referred by family physicians, at the physician's office, and supports an average of four family physicians. The home care nurse provides care according to algorithms, tracks care using the Region's chronic disease management information system, admits patients with chronic disease to home care, maintains links with specialist clinicians and with regional/community programmes, and carries out one-to-one telephone follow-up with patients. Family physicians may invoice Alberta Health and Wellness for these services. Nurse case managers receive additional chronic disease and case management training (Delon 2006).

education, follow-up and transfer to primary care practices; clinical practice guidelines embedded in documents to assist clinicians in providing standardized evidence-based guidelines to patients; alerts and reminders to ensure compliance with clinical practice guidelines and patient safety/health issues; and continuous documentation of patient health information once enrolled on a pathway (Donaldson-Kelly 2007). The chronic disease management strategies in Calgary Health Region include specialist expertise; nurse case management (Box 9.2); an electronic chronic disease information system; and a Living Well with a Chronic Condition self-management programme (Calgary Health Region 2007).

The Alberta NetCare Electronic Health Record is a province-wide health information system that links physicians, pharmacists, hospitals, home care and other providers across the province (Alberta NetCare 2007). The electronic health record stores pertinent patient information online to allow health care providers instant electronic access to a patient's prescription history, allergies and laboratory results. Both Calgary and Edmonton health regions have invested in regional portals that integrate data from various sources (Box 9.3). Alberta has focused on disease-specific minimum data sets. Physician involvement has been negligible to date.

> **Box 9.3 Electronic Health Record system (NetCare) in Edmonton health region**
>
> Capital Health's Electronic Health Record system (NetCare) was rolled out across the region in 2004 (Capital Health Electronic Health Record 2004), providing instant access to medical records. Focusing, for example, on diabetes patients, the system compiles comprehensive clinical information that registers and tracks diabetic patients. It includes standardized workflow consistent with clinical practice guidelines; monitoring of minimum data sets; decision support for providers with recommendations and reminders; standardized reporting; and updating of forms as required. Key information from the electronic medical records is posted on the Alberta Electronic Health Record system NetCare. NetCare data are available to the Diabetes Centre Team, primary care providers, hospital emergency departments, after-hours clinics, pharmacies, and community home care teams.

In **Quebec**, there has been an ongoing effort to enhance accessible, comprehensive, continuous and coordinated care for people with complex needs, including those with chronic disease. Two recent reforms have been of particular importance: the reorganization in 2003 of Quebec's health and social service network into local service networks (CSSS) and the introduction of family medicine groups (FMGs) from 2002 in an attempt to ensure comprehensive and continuous case management to meet the population's health and social care needs (Box 9.4). Another key initiative is the Programme to Integrate Information Services and Manage Education (PRIISME). It uses

---

Box 9.4 Health and social services centres and family medicine groups in Quebec

Health and social services centres (CSSS) in Quebec are mandated to (1) provide a comprehensive package of services to a defined population, including prevention, assessment, diagnosis, treatment, adjustment, integration, rehabilitation, residential care and end-of-life support; (2) introduce care models that ensure comprehensive, ongoing and personalized case management; (3) create conditions that foster continuity of care; and (4) develop intersectoral cooperation to create living environments conducive to the population's health. The CSSS bring together the local community health centres (CLSCs), residential and long-term care centres (CHSLDs) and the community hospitals within a given territory. They develop partnerships essential to the operation of the networks, particularly with physicians, community organizations, private medical clinics and intersectoral resources. The implementation of the CSSS is well under way in the different regions of Quebec and the different components of the network complement each other to provide a more comprehensive set of services to particular clienteles. The main challenge for the years to come will still be to increase coordination between these different components.

Family medicine groups (FMGs) in Quebec are very similar to Ontario's Family Health Teams (FHTs). An FMG brings together 6 to 12 GPs who commit to providing a full range of medical case management services and extended hours to patients who have chosen to enrol with them. Services include patient assessment, care and follow-up, diagnosis and treatment of acute and chronic problems, along with disease prevention and health promotion. These services are provided 24 hours a day, 7 days a week. FMGs services are intended to complement those provided by CLSCs, hospitals and emergency departments. They increasingly make use of nursing staff to support physicians in the different stages of the care process.

Montreal Region also developed so-called associate medical centres (AMC) (Agence de Développement des Réseaux Locaux de Santé et de Services Sociaux de Montréal 2004). AMCs aim to ensure operational coordination between the physicians in a given territory and the CSSS. An AMC may be a clinic, a group of clinics, a medical team of a CLSC, an FMG or a family medicine unit. AMCs have to meet a set of conditions: (1) coordinate and liaise with the local CSSS; (2) provide a full range of front-line medical services seven days a week; (3) guarantee medical after-hour services for at-risk patients; (4) coordinate medical services and ensure liaison with the relevant CSSS; (5) provide local GPs with appropriate technical support for diagnostic tests; and (6) provide services according to a comprehensive, continuous and personalized approach (50% of activities must be devoted to medical follow-up appointments to obtain the AMC status from the regional agency).

a comprehensive approach, integrating the main steps involved in patient management, including prevention, diagnosis, treatment, drug compliance and follow-up. Centred on self-management, the programme builds on a primary care model and promotes an interdisciplinary approach. Since 1999, PRIISME has implemented more than 25 projects in Quebec, focusing on asthma, COPD and diabetes, along with other projects developed in Ontario. Key strategies include concerted efforts by RHAs and/or the provincial government, institutions, community groups, private medical clinics and health professionals; continuing education for all health professionals, including physicians, nurses and pharmacists; and disease management education for patients and their families. Quebec has also been experimenting with new models of care developed from major research initiatives such as the System of Integrated Services for the Frail Elderly (SIPA) and the Program of Research to Integrate the Services for the Maintenance of Autonomy (PRISMA) that focus on integrated networks and interprofessional collaboration to improve care for those with complex needs (Bergman et al. 1997, Hébert et al. 2003).

Chronic disease management in Ontario

Ontario has a history of chronic disease initiatives at provincial, municipal and community levels. A 2004 study identified 159 chronic disease management teams in Ontario, 110 of which had been in place for at least three years, although only few programmes covered the entire range of assessment, diagnosis, treatment, education and follow-up (The Change Foundation 2004). At present, Ontario has numerous small- and large-scale chronic disease prevention strategies and programmes but these services are generally fragmented and substantially underfunded (Ontario Chronic Disease Prevention Alliance 2006). More recently, there has been a growing emphasis on improving governance and management of chronic diseases by the provincial government, health networks and community organizations. The current Ontario government has made a commitment to keep people healthy and has developed a number of strategies since the early 2000s impacting on prevention and chronic disease management. These include the introduction of a Ministry of Health Promotion, family health teams (FHTs), and LHINs.

The Ministry of Health Promotion has a population health focus and has, together with the Ontario Ministry of Health and Long-Term Care, developed major provincial strategies targeting tobacco use, stroke, cancer, osteoporosis and diabetes, as well as Ontario's Chronic Disease Prevention and Management (CDPM) framework (Ontario Chronic Disease Prevention Alliance 2006). The CDPM framework has formed the basis for a range of activities, including recommendations for shifting FHTs to focus on chronic disease management;

the expansion of the provincial government's Asthma Strategy and the recent Diabetes Strategy focusing on diabetes education, early intervention and effective prevention of complications. Regional planning and implementation of CDPM is through LHINs. The Ontario government has also invested in IT to create a central electronic health records database. Furthermore, through Telehealth Ontario, residents have access to a registered nurse 24 hours a day, 7 days a week for health-related queries and concerns.

FHTs were implemented across the province since 2004 as part of Ontario's health transformation agenda to promote patient-centred, integrated health care, reduce waiting times and increase access. FHTs are to provide comprehensive, coordinated, interdisciplinary primary care services to a defined population on a round-the-clock basis with physicians working as a part of a team involving nurse practitioners, mental health care staff and social workers. The core services provided by FHTs include health promotion and disease prevention, chronic disease management and self-management support. Patient enrolment with an FHT physician is voluntary; incentives for physicians to participate in the scheme include choice of governance model, blended compensation, working in interdisciplinary teams, and flexibility to meet population needs. However, it is not known at the time of writing whether all FHTs are operating according to the intended interdisciplinary model as no systematic evaluation has been carried out thus far.

From 2005, Ontario has also begun to regionalize community health care, through the establishment of 14 LHINs. LHINs are tasked with planning, coordinating and funding health services through agreements with health care providers such as hospitals and home care organizations (for example, long-term care institutions and Community Care Access Centres). Several LHINs have included chronic disease management and prevention as a priority area. Most LHINs have now developed a working group or strategies to work collaboratively with primary care providers.

In the subsection that follows we describe cancer care as an example of a structured disease management programme in Ontario.

Cancer Care Ontario

Until 2004, cancer services in Ontario were characterized by fragmentation and complexity, with inequalities in access to services, supportive care, health information and palliative care (Canadian Cancer Society and CCO 2003, Sullivan et al. 2003). For example, between 1997 and 2004, outpatient cancer treatment was provided at 11 Regional Cancer Centres operated by Cancer Care Ontario (CCO), a freestanding agency under the auspices of the Ontario Ministry of Health and Long-Term Care, and located in either academic medical centres or major regional tertiary facilities, with the remaining services being provided by teaching and community hospitals, community clinics, physicians, voluntary organizations, and Community Care Access Centres.

In an attempt to move towards a more integrated approach to cancer services, CCO shifted from being a direct provider of services to focusing on providing strategic leadership and driving quality of and access to care in 2004. The 11 Regional Cancer Centres that were previously operated by CCO were integrated with their host hospitals, thus creating 14 Regional Cancer Programs that align with LHINs. CCO has become the main organization responsible for the overall cancer system strategy, including planning, establishing standards and guidelines, measuring and reporting on the performance of the cancer system at local and provincial levels, purchasing some services, conducting and disseminating research, and innovation. It acts as chief advisor to the Ontario Ministry of Health and Long-Term Care on cancer care and services. The 14 Regional Cancer Programs are virtual programmes that link cancer providers, community organizations, patients and decision-makers across the full spectrum of cancer care, including prevention, screening, diagnosis, treatment, and supportive and palliative care (CCO 2005a). Regional Cancer Programs develop work plans that address local priorities and provincial initiatives. Each Regional Cancer Program has an appointed Regional Vice-President (RVP) for cancer services who is accountable to both CCO and the host hospital. RVPs manage the Regional Cancer Programs, advise CCO on regional issues, build and strengthen community partnerships to coordinate planning at regional levels and work towards improving regional performance as measured by cancer care performance indicators. There are also regional clinical leaders assigned to each domain of the care continuum (such as screening, surgical oncology, family medicine) who participate in the Regional Cancer Programs.

Health system features supporting programmes

Given the variety of programmes targeting chronic disease across Canada, this section focuses more specifically on health system features supporting chronic disease management in Ontario, in some instances using CCO as an example.

Targets, standards and guidelines

CCO is an example of one of the most detailed and specific plans for addressing a single, but complex, chronic disease. Using the Ontario Cancer Registry (OCR) and clinical administrative data, CCO developed a comprehensive cancer plan for Ontario that is the first of its kind in Canada. The *Ontario Cancer Plan 2005–2008* addresses the growing demand for cancer services, looking 10 years into the future, with a detailed action plan for the first three years. This plan was based on *Cancer 2020 Targeting Cancer: An action plan for cancer prevention and detection,* which details specific goals, targets and recommendations for prevention and detection (Canadian Cancer Society and CCO 2003).

CCO supports leadership and partnership through the development of evidence-based standards and guidelines to help clinicians across the continuum of care to keep up with new clinical information. It has developed a Program in Evidence-Based Care which synthesizes and reviews research evidence and develops practice guidelines. CCO has also developed a palliative care strategy. Various CCO clinical programmes and peer groups come together to share best practices. Mechanisms for knowledge brokering include sharing best practices, reviewing indicator data, workshops and Communities of Practice (Sawka 2005). CCO is involved in the systematic collection, storage, access and use of information with its partners.

CCO has also implemented a fully-automated cancer drug ordering system that includes clinical guidelines, safety information, and pharmaceutical utilization information, available through an adapted model of Computerized Physician Order Entry (CPOE). The Pathology Information Management System (PIMS) facilitates tracking of each patient's passage through the system (CCO 2005a). In 2006, an information system was developed that would lead to the creation of an electronic health record. By December 2006, the Wait Time Information Strategy Enterprise Master Patient Index had been implemented in 53 hospitals, accounting for 90% of the five priority procedures (cancer surgeries, cataract surgeries, hip and knee replacement, and magnetic resonance imaging (MRI) and computed tomography (CT) scans) (CCO 2007b).

As part of the strategy to address quality issues, in 2002 the Ministry of Health established a Cancer Quality Council of Ontario with a mandate to monitor and report on key indicators of cancer system performance. In April 2005, the Council released a Cancer System Quality Index (CQSI) comprising 25 measures of quality. This helps to track the quality and consistency of key services delivered across Ontario's cancer system, from prevention to end-of-life care (CCO 2005a).

One of the key challenges in chronic disease management is how to ensure clinical accountability. In the case of CCO, this is done via two main routes. First, accountability is ensured through quarterly reporting, joint review meetings to discuss significant performance issues, and production of performance improvement plans. The regional vice-presidents work with hospitals and other providers to address issues that arise and they regularly report on the progress of their regional centres at community forums and in community partnership meetings. Information from the CQSI is used to identify areas that are working well and those that need improvement.

A second, complementary route involves financial incentives. In Ontario, hospitals are funded through a global budget. CCO funds Regional Cancer Centres which are incorporated with host hospitals and provides funding to hospitals for new investments in cancer care. This funding is linked to a comprehensive agreement with hospitals that sets out joint accountability for quality improvement, treatment volumes (jointly agreed), and access to hospital data. These include standardized pathology reporting, use of cancer staging guidelines, regular reports on the care of each patient following discharge, and provision of data on waiting times for cancer surgery. In 2006, CCO allocated CAD 27 million (€18.4 million) of government funding to the hospitals to deliver 11% (or 4817) more cancer operations, with the aim of reducing waiting times (CCO 2005a).

In addition, there are financial incentives (in the form of salary supplements) built into the system for medical and radiation oncologists in order to increase time dedicated to patient encounters as a means of improving quality of care.

Health care workforce and capacity

Human resources remain a major challenge in Ontario, given insufficient numbers of appropriately trained personnel (especially pathologists and radiologists) for present and future needs in hospitals and the community. The ageing population contributes to increased incidence of chronic diseases, requiring multi-skilled professionals with new competencies. An Ontario Medical Association study released in November 2005 reported that the physician workforce is shrinking. A total of 19% of practising physicians are over 60 years and 11% are over 65 years (Ontario Medical Association 2005). More trained professionals undertaking innovative new roles are needed in order to address this problem. In May 2006 the Ontario government announced an investment of CAD 45 million (€30.6 million) in *HealthForceOntario* to create new and innovative roles such as physician assistants and nurse endoscopists, and to expand training programmes for physicians, pharmacists and nurses (Ministry of Health Welfare and Sport 2006).

Evaluation and lessons learned

Ontario provides a good example of the substantial challenges faced by a government that is attempting to reform its health system, moving from a model focused on acute care to an integrated patient-centred health system, with the difficulties highlighted by a recent assessment by the Ontario Health

Quality Council (Ontario Health Quality Council 2007). This shift requires critical elements of infrastructure, such as a clinical information system with patient registers, decision support and self-management support. The Ontario government's 2004 transformation agenda included an e-health strategy, interdisciplinary family health networks and regionalized health organizations (LHINs), as described earlier. However, the FHTs and LHINs are unable to function adequately without an electronic health record system, and progress on e-health in Ontario has been painfully slow.

Ontario is performing poorly in terms of self-management support for patients with chronic conditions. Several organizations offer self-management support, such as Community Health Centres or associations such as Arthritis Canada (Box 9.5). In Ontario, one of the key objectives of the FHT is to provide self-management care as part of their disease management activities, and there is a commitment in the Physician's Service Agreement 2004 – negotiated with the Ontario Medical Association – that the Ontario Ministry of Health and Long-Term Care will identify appropriate support materials for the primary health care sector and distribute it to enrolled patients. Additionally, the CDPM sub-committee of the FHT Action Group, an advisory group for the health transformation initiative, identified self-management as an important area for further action. Self-management is also an integral component in the guide to chronic disease management for FHTs that has been developed by the provincial health ministry (Ontario Ministry of Health and Long-Term Care 2005). However, there has been no evaluation of whether this is being implemented and overall it appears that structured support to patients remains underdeveloped, with recent figures suggesting that, for example, only 28% of people with diabetes have access to structured diabetes education (Ontario Health Quality Council 2007). High rates of readmission to hospitals also point to poor management of chronic disease overall. For example, in Ontario, one in seven newly diagnosed patients with heart failure is readmitted to hospital within 90 days of discharge (Lee, Joahnsen & Gong 2004).

Box 9.5 Supporting cancer patients in Ontario

Many hospitals in Ontario that have Regional Cancer Programs offer structured support to patients and their families, although the nature of that support varies. For example, Toronto Sunnybrook Regional Cancer Centre has developed a special support programme enabling its cancer patients to obtain treatment on an outpatient basis; it includes nutrition and psychological counselling, social worker assistance and support groups. The Canadian Cancer Association provides a variety of patient support programmes, including trained volunteers providing home support. The largest gap in patient support remains in hospitals that are not Regional Cancer Centres, where the nearest cancer centre may be geographically distant, as is the case in many rural areas.

Until recently, Ontario, unlike the rest of Canada, did not have a regionalized health care model. The establishment of LHINs is therefore being undertaken in phases, with LHINs expected to become fully functional during 2008. The Ontario Ministry of Health and Long-Term care also needed to reform its bureaucracy in order to meet the evolving needs of LHINs, and to reflect the Ministry's new "stewardship role" (Ontario Ministry of Health and Long-Term Care 2007). It has established a Chronic Disease Unit to implement the CDPM.

Ontario's health care system faces serious capacity problems, with Ontario having one of the lowest ratios of physicians per population in Canada, as well as a shortage of nurses and an increasing burden of disease as a result of an ageing population. The shortage of physicians arose for many reasons, including a decrease in the number of international medical graduates, a significant decrease in medical school enrolments, along with retirement. The FHTs are being implemented in this challenging environment. While FHT guidelines for chronic disease management propose that physicians provide support for self-management to patients, it is questionable how this may be possible in the current situation. Short-term disease-specific approaches are not able to adapt to the rapidly changing chronic disease environment. In summary, the Ontario government has developed a chronic disease framework for multiple strategies, but, at the time of writing, it is only implementing a Diabetes Strategy, with the expectation that appropriate infrastructure could be developed in the near future to implement other chronic disease strategies.

Cancer Care Ontario

Available evidence suggests a good standard of care for those diagnosed with cancer. According to the 2007 Cancer Quality Index, progress has been made on several indicators including: smoking rates, the continued decline of which has been attributed to Ontario's comprehensive Smoke-Free Ontario strategy; improved survival for patients with the three of the four most common cancers (prostate, breast and colorectal); support for evidence-based care (42 new guidelines in 2006); and high uptake of CCO's Computerized Physician Order Entry system (CCO 2007a).

CCO has, however, recognized that it needs to pay more attention to the continuum of care, including prevention, screening, diagnosis and palliative care (CCO 2006). Previously, CCO's focus had been largely on diagnosis and treatment, with little attention to education and support for self-management by patients. More recently this focus has shifted, with the development of web-based information on prevention and screening for key cancer types, such as breast, cervical and colorectal cancers. In addition, recognizing screening as an effective way of reducing the burden of disease for some types of cancer, CCO has, in partnership with the Ontario Ministry of Health and Long-Term Care, committed to implement a province-wide colorectal screening programme. However, the Ontario government has not endorsed the Cancer 2020 Plan, which targets prevention and detection (PCPSC 2006).

CCO has made considerable progress in other areas, including developing new professional roles, such as nurse-performed flexible sigmoidoscopy and advanced practice radiation therapists, as part of the *HealthForceOntario* plan, as well as facilitating knowledge development and exchange by enhanced training of health professionals.

From a system perspective, CCO provides insights into how a government agency responsible for a single disease has utilized various levers to improve quality of care and to facilitate partnerships among disparate health service organizations, professionals, decision-makers and patients, so as to improve the patient journey. Some of the key identifiable best practices within CCO are listed here.

- A targeted plan with clear goals and outcomes, including public reporting of progress. For example, investment priorities for 2007–2010 include standards and guidelines, performance measurement and accountability, and rapid access strategies.

- An information management and IT plan and strategies (that is, IM/IT Strategic Plan 2008–2011 (CCO 2008)), to enhance the capacity of CCO and other providers to deliver quality cancer services.

- Joint accountability for quality of care between providers and central organization.

- A combination of strategies to ensure continuous quality improvement and organizational excellence, such as development of regional accountability mechanisms, with sanctions for underperformance; a "pay for performance" strategy to improve the quality of care; quality improvement targeting the entire continuum of care, and involving planners, health service providers, and government policy-makers; influencing clinical outcomes through Communities of Practice, peer-to-peer education, and the use of evidence-based guidelines; and using credible evidence-based data to influence change management.

Investing in the future

This chapter describes a wide range of individual initiatives, from across Canada's provinces and territories. Many include elements that look ahead to future needs, building in the flexibility that is needed for future proofing. It gives examples of how the various actors have reacted to problems emerging

Table 9.1 *Cancer Care Ontario: strengths and weaknesses*

	Strengths	Weaknesses	Opportunities	Threats
Central agency governance model	Acts as a champion of quality–outcome of care Strong focus on specific areas of management of the system, e.g. evidence-based guidelines, performance management, and information management Central leadership in promoting partnerships/linkages, and provincial-level planning Capacity for driving innovation change management	Limited benefits to regions that do not have regional programmes Can only be effective in health system areas that it is responsible for Lack of clear distinction of responsibilities in many areas of its current work in terms of the roles of physician/hospital associations, LHINs, and the Ministry of Health	Redefinition of the role of CCO within the new LHIN structure (LHINs have regional planning and coordinating responsibilities, and accountability for hospitals) Evaluation of the effectiveness of the CCO agency model with the potential of knowledge transfer to management of chronic diseases from a system perspective	Potential of centralization of power within a single agency that may pose challenges to certain areas of system integration for chronic diseases Potential conflict of roles between CCO, LHINs, hospitals, physician associations, and the Ministry of Health Variation in regional access

(cont.)

Table 9.1 *(cont.)*

	Strengths	Weaknesses	Opportunities	Threats
Integrated patient-centred care	Provides an alternative/innovative model of addressing some of the key components of integrated care, e.g. coordination, partnership, decision support	Acute care focus	Redefinition of the role of CCO within the new regionalized structure	Series of patient encounters in continuity of care with no central coordination for assessment, support or follow-up
		Lack of structured patient education or self-management support for survivors		
	Facilitation of patient journey from treatment to palliative care	Weak prevention efforts but making some progress	Lessons can be learnt from evaluating this model from an integrated system perspective to improve chronic care	General weaknesses of the Ontario health system, e.g. lack of primary electronic medical records, waiting times for diagnosis, rising obesity rates
	Active role in prevention efforts through screening and early detection for certain types of cancer	Fragmented care for cancer patients, e.g. those within CCO regional cancer programmes and those that are non-CCO patients		How to promote equitable/integrated care without losing key CCO roles that have improved cancer care

Source: Authors' own compilation.

Note: LHIN: Local Health Integration Networks; CCO: Cancer Care Ontario.

at different levels, such as the major investment in training of physicians in Ontario, in the face of looming shortages. Ontario's government has used the federal Primary Health Care Transition Fund to enhance access to primary health care; establish interdisciplinary primary care teams; and increase the emphasis on health promotion, disease and injury prevention, and management of chronic diseases.

The approach to cancer care is illustrative. The Ontario government has made substantial investments to increase the capacity of cancer services, including facility expansion and equipment acquisition, with an emphasis on reducing waiting times for surgery. This included a commitment in 2004 of CAD 26.3 million (€17.9 million) to improve cancer care across the province. Approximately CAD 15 million (€10.2 million) was earmarked to improve access, and CAD 10 million (€6.8 million) to reduce waiting times for surgery and diagnostic services (CCO 2005b). The Ontario government has also created the Ontario Institute for Cancer Research to advance research in cancer prevention, diagnosis and treatment.

The approach taken by CCO is set out in Table 9.1. The organization has focused on a few key areas, using a variety of levers to promote change. Moving forward from the gains made in many areas of cancer care in the province since its first strategic plan in 2004, CCO has now developed a strategic plan for 2008–2011 that includes increasing cancer screening through vigorous education and screening strategies, and providing tools to assist physicians and patients to participate in screening, including using IT proficiently to send out invitations, reminders and prompts about screening. Such techniques are important in the management of cancer and other chronic diseases.

References

Agence de Développement des Réseaux Locaux de Santé et de Services Sociaux de Montréal (2004). *The organization of front-line medical services in Montreal, CSSS René-Cassin et NDG/Montréal-Ouest*. Montreal, Agence de Développement des Réseaux Locaux de Santé et de Services Sociaux de Montréal.

Alberta NetCare (2007). Alberta NetCare information [web site]. Edmonton, Alberta NetCare (http://www.albertanetcare.ca/2.htm, accessed 13 August 2008).

Bergman H et al. (1997). Care for Canada's frail elderly population: fragmentation or integration. *Canadian Medical Association Journal*, 157:1116–1121.

Calgary Health Region (2007) [web site]. Chronic disease management. Calgary, Calgary Health Region (http://www.calgaryhealthregion.ca/cdm/index.html, accessed 13 August 2008).

Canadian Cancer Society & CCO (2003). *Targeting cancer: An action plan for cancer prevention and detection*. Toronto, Cancer Care Ontario, Canadian Cancer Society (Cancer 2020 summary report).

CCO (2005a). *Ontario Cancer Plan: 2005 progress report*. Toronto, Cancer Care Ontario.

CCO (2005b). Cancer Care Ontario in the news [web site]. Toronto, Cancer Care Ontario (http://www.cancercare.on.ca/OntarioCancerNewsArchives/200503/index_404.htm, accessed 13 August 2008).

CCO (2006) [web site]. Cancer system quality index 2006. Toronto, Cancer Care Ontario (http://www.cancercare.on.ca/qualityindex2006/, accessed 6 May 2008).

CCO (2007a). Cancer system quality index 2007 [web site]. Toronto, Cancer Care Ontario (http://www.cancercare.on.ca/qualityindex2007/, accessed 6 May 2008).

CCO (2007b). *Ontario Cancer Plan: 2006–2007 progress report. Building a patient-centered cancer system across Ontario*. Toronto, Cancer Care Ontario.

CCO (2008). IM/IT strategic plan 2008–2011 [web site]. Toronto, Cancer Care Ontario (http://www.cancercare.on.ca/english/home/about/initiatives/imstrategy/, accessed May 2008).

Capital Health Electronic Record (2004). Capital Health's new electronic health record rolls out across the region. *Capital Health Quarterly*, Winter/Spring:6–7.

CCDPC (2007) [web site]. The Canadian Best Practices Portal for Health Promotion and Chronic Disease Prevention. Ottawa, Public Health Agency of Canada (http://cbpp-pcpe.phac-aspc.gc.ca/, accessed 13 August 2008).

Church J, Barker P (1998). Regionalization of health services in Canada: A critical perspective. *International Journal of Health Services*, 28:467–486.

Dallhousie University (2003). *Nova Scotia Chronic Disease Prevention Strategy*. Halifax, Dalhousie University, Unit for Population Health and Chronic Disease Prevention (on behalf of Working Group Members).

Delon S (2006). *Chronic disease management: Calgary Health Region*. Ontario, Southwestern Ontario Regional Partnership Leadership Forum (www.lhsc.on.ca/isan/projects/sworp/2006_Pres/SWO_RegPrtnrshp_news_Fall06.pdf, accessed 6 May 2008).

Denis JL (2002). *Gouvernance et gestion du changement dans le système de santé au Canada*. Ottawa, Commission on the future of health care in Canada.

Donaldson-Kelly S (2007). Personal communication. Stephanie Donaldson Kelly, Director of Operations, Chronic Disease Management, Capital Health.

Government of British Columbia Ministry of Health (2007) [web site]. Chronic disease management. Victoria, Ministry of Health of the Government of British Columbia (http://www.health.gov.bc.ca/cdm/index.html, accessed 13 August 2008).

Health Council of Canada (2007). *Why health care renewal matters. Lessons from diabetes*. Toronto, Health Council of Canada.

Health Quality Council (2005). Saskatchewan Chronic Disease Management Collaborative [web site]. Saskatoon, Health Quality Council (http://www.hqc.sk.ca/portal.jsp?CdSpcZ7g0/9pTSydwUWU7jBIzBf0QfLQkUwK4QBZaJvwO9ghh5dfuYzOVcA+lmY4, accessed 13 August 2008).

Hébert R et al. (2003). PRISMA: a new model of integrated service delivery for the frail older people in Canada. *International Journal of Integrated Care*, 3:e08.

Lee DS, Johansen H, Gong Y (2004). Regional outcome of heart failure in Canada. In: Tu JV, Ghali WA, Pilote L (eds). *Canadian cardiovascular atlas*. Toronto, Institute for Clinical Evaluative Sciences:111–119.

Marchildon GP (2005). Health systems in transition: Canada. *Health Systems in Transition*, 7(3):1–156.

Ministry of Health Welfare and Sport (2006). *Wet Maatschappelijke Ondersteuning. Iedereen moet mee kunnen doen [Act on Social Support, everybody should be able to participate]*. The Hague, Netherlands Ministry of Health, Welfare and Sport.

Ontario Chronic Disease Prevention Alliance (2006). *Thinking like a system: The way forward to prevent chronic disease in Ontario*. Toronto, Ontario Chronic Disease Alliance.

Ontario Health Quality Council (2007). *Report on Ontario's health system*. Toronto, Ontario Health Quality Council.

Ontario Medical Association (2005). *The Ontario physician shortage 2005: seeds of progress, but resource crisis deepening*. Toronto, Ontario Medical Association (http://www.oma.org/pcomm/OMR/nov/05physicianshortage.htm, accessed 13 August 2008) (OMA Position Paper).

Ontario Ministry of Health and Long-Term Care (2005). *Family health teams: A guide to chronic disease management and prevention*. Toronto, Ontario Ministry of Health and Long-Term Care.

Ontario Ministry of Health and Long-Term Care (2007). *Local health integration networks*. Bulletin 25. Toronto, Ontario Ministry of Health and Long-Term Care (http://www.health.gov.on.ca/transformation/lhin/20070208/lhin_bul_25_20070208.html, accessed 13 August 2008).

PCPSC (2006). Approved minutes from meeting, 26 February. Toronto, Cancer Care Ontario Provincial Cancer Prevention and Screening Council. (www.cancercare.on/documents/PCPSC-Minutes24Feb2006_Approved.pdf, accessed 13 August 2008).

Sawka C (2005). *Using guidelines and accountability strategies to improve patient outcomes*. Toronto, Ontario Hospital Association HealthAchieve (https://ospace.scholarsportal.info/bitstream/1873/2123/1/259119.pdf, accessed 15 August 2008).

Sullivan T et al. (2003). *Strengthening the quality of cancer services in Ontario*. Ottawa, Canadian Healthcare Association Press.

The Change Foundation (2004). *Seeking program sustainability in chronic disease management: The Ontario experience*. Toronto, The Change Foundation.

Secretariat for the Intersectoral Healthy Living Network, in partnership with the F/P/T Healthy Living Task Group & the F/P/T Advisory Committee on Population Health and Health Security (2005). *The integrated pan-Canadian healthy living strategy*. Ottawa, Canadian Minister of Health.

WHIC (2006) [web site]. About WHIC. Edmonton, Western Health Information Collaborative (http://www.whic.org/, accessed 13 August 2008).